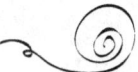

Slugs Don't Eat Arugula

*Tales of Whimsy, Woe, and Wisdom
from the Kitchen and Garden*

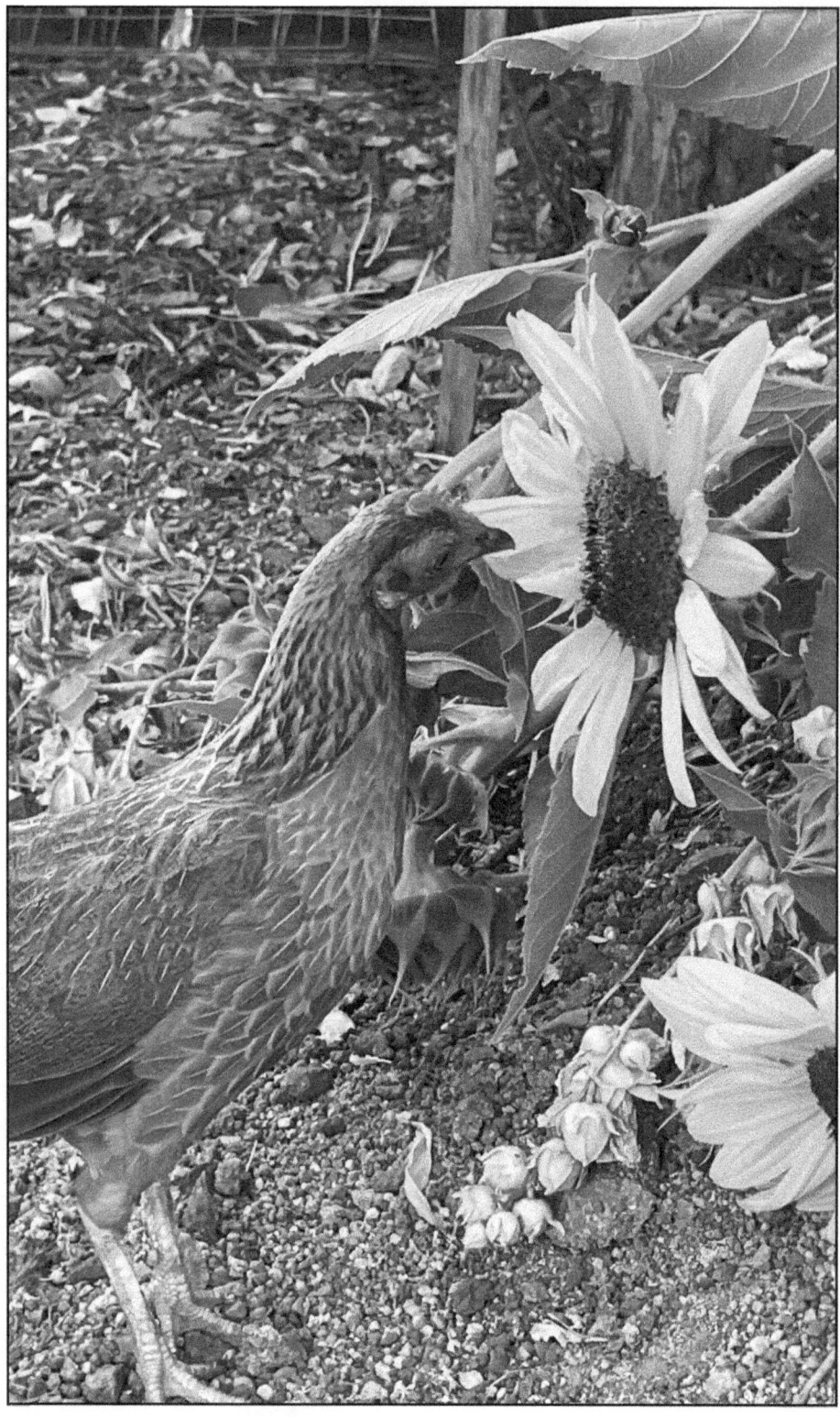

Slugs Don't Eat Arugula

Tales of Whimsy, Woe, and Wisdom from the Kitchen and Garden

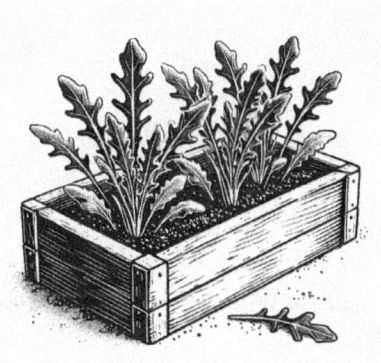

JEREMY MILLER

Memoir Books
Chico, California

Slugs Don't Eat Arugula: Tales of Whimsy, Woe, and Wisdom from the Kitchen and Garden

Copyright ©2025 by Jeremy Miller
ISBN: 978-1-937748-43-2
Library of Congress Control Number: 2025905821

All rights reserved. No portion of this book may be used for any AI purposes, reproduced, or reprinted in any manner whatsoever (except in reviews) that is in violation of copyright restrictions without written permission.

Artwork: DALL·E and Google emojis
Front cover photograph by Earl Bloor with additional photo editing by Maxx Hill.

Layout/design by Josie Reifschneider-Smith, Heidelberg Graphics

Memoir Books, *an Imprint of Heidelberg Graphics*, Chico, CA, USA
HeidelbergGraphics@gmail.com

Contents

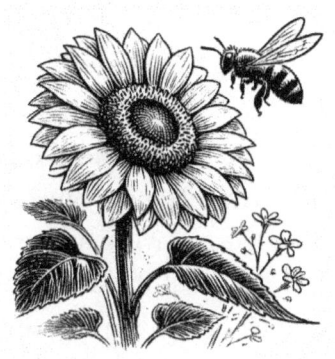

Author's Note and Acknowledgements
vi

Kitchen Conundrums and Recipes for Disaster
1

In Search of the Green Thumb
19

Overland Migratory Gophers (OMGs) & Other Critters
41

Food Forest Follies
61

Food on the Go
74

The Witch Doctor's Pantry
83

Kettle Chips Are My Kryptonite
92

Feed Your Soul
108

Author's Note & Acknowledgements

Most of these essays appeared as earlier drafts in *Edible Shasta-Butte* magazine beginning in 2011. They are organized in this book by topic and flow, like a playlist, and are not in chronological order. As such, the reader will note that the diet choices of my family are not fully consistent from chapter to chapter, and similarly the age of my daughters varies widely. For those who wish to know, the chapter, "Kettle Chips Are My Kryptonite" describes the most recent eating habits of my family (as of spring 2024), and at the time this book went to press my daughters were 16 and 13 years old.

The creation of this book was not a one-person job. I would first and foremost like to thank Candace Bryne and the late Earl Bloor, editors emeriti of Edible Shasta-Butte magazine, for providing me with a platform where I could share my musings over the years, as well as to the many readers of said magazine who warmly expressed their appreciation for my efforts. Earl also took the photo that graces the front of this book; graphic designer Maxx Hill provided addtional photo-editing. I extend my gratitude to Scott Wolf, Mike Graf, and Irene Salter, fellow authors and friends who provided timely advice which helped me to move this project forward. I would like to thank my family for their continued support of my creative side, including my wife Amy who served as both wordsmith and proofreader for many early versions of these essays, and to my daughters Zia and Tali (who grace the front and back covers respectively), for their joyful roles in the stories found here-in. OpenAI's open-source text-to-image model DALL-E 3 was utilized to create the art that appears throughout the book. Lastly, I wish to acknowledge the efforts of my editor, Josie Reifschneider-Smith, who worked diligently with me to bring this project to its current form.

To the reader: Delight in the feasts both small and large, the spontaneous bouquets, the sun and the rain, the bees, and all the joys that come from the garden and the kitchen. —JM

CHAPTER 1

Kitchen Conundrums and Recipes for Disaster

Kale Chips

I was first introduced to kale chips at an upscale restaurant in the San Francisco Bay Area. Fried in olive oil with a hint of salt, two chips were laid delicately over a bed of mashed Yukon Gold potatoes. They were melt-in-your-mouth divine, like green, super-thin potato chips from heaven, only pretending to be healthier. So when I first saw a bag of kale chips for sale in a store, it was a no-think impulse buy, despite the $3.99 price tag for two ounces of food. The purchase turned out to be a disappointment. Once opened, the package revealed cold, fossilized leaves of kale that were encrusted with flakes of "cheese" and seasoned with assorted spices. While the oil and salt appealed to my primal side, the semi-soapy texture of the cheese made it impossible to finish the bag.

Then my brother told me about making kale chips at home. "No, thank you," I replied. I could turn a blind eye to the grease present in the package of chips, but deep-frying anything at home crossed the health line for me. "You don't understand," he said. "You just toss the kale leaves lightly with some olive oil and salt and then bake them. It is really good." I was skeptical, but this message—and recipe—were repeated to me by no fewer than three friends over the next few months, usually while I was surveying the fresh produce at the farmers' market.

Kale is a terrific vegetable, and it is the perfect winter green. It is flavorful; has a longer shelf life in the refrigerator as compared to other greens; and is rich in antioxidants and vitamins C, K, and A. (Confession: I don't really know what antioxidants are, but they sound healthy thanks to the artful marketing of the nutrition industry.)

While you can find kale pretty much year round, the best season in my region is the frosty months, when the leaves are milder and the aphids are on vacation. In the middle of winter, I can go to the farmers' market and choose from no fewer than five varieties of kale of varying textures and shades of green and purple, often for a just a couple bucks a bundle. All taste wonderful. I have had great success with quickly sautéing kale on high heat in some oil with garlic or sneaking some chopped leaves into a stew. Others rave about shredded raw kale salads, garnished with carrot slivers, salted sunflower seeds, and raisins.

Some sound advice for making kale chips: the thicker the leaf, the better the chip. But beyond this, I recommend the reader seek counsel elsewhere. After my first attempt, the baking sheet looked like the aftermath of a brush fire, with an occasional tuft of green poking through the charcoal remains. A couple weeks later I tried again. This time the result was a mosaic of brown and green and looked about as appetizing as dry leaves on a compost heap, which, coincidentally, is what it became. For my last try it was wilt city: The once perky foliage looked as if it had been drained of its life by vegetarian vampires, but at least the leaves were still green.

At this point you might logically ask: "What recipe were you using?" The answer: All of them. When you type "How to make kale chips" into your web browser, the first five recipes give oven temperatures ranging from 250-350F degrees, and a cooking time of anywhere from 8 to 35 minutes. Throw in the fact that my oven's internal thermometer has the reliability of a weather forecaster (it takes me well over an hour to bake a 40-minute banana bread), my chances of success were grim indeed.

But let's call a spade a spade—the next time you want to ramble on about kale chips, know that the real reason you like them is because of the olive oil and salt.

Kitchen Superhero Utility Belt

If I had a superhero utility belt for my time in the kitchen, it would hold four must-have items: a serrated paring knife, a spatula, a chainmail scrubber, and a wooden spoon.

The paring knife, of course, is the most essential. Over the course of an hour on a standard weekday morning, I use my knife to slice and core an apple, trim greens, butter toast, cut sausage, and dice cucumbers, bell peppers, and onion for a side salad. Yes, I do rinse the knife in between uses—I'm not a complete troglodyte—though I do admit to drying it on my terry cloth apron.

Adjacent to the knife is the spatula. Mine is a Richcraft 14-inch Stainless Steel Slotted Spatula, model #4015S (with a phoenix feather core). It performs the usual tasks admirably: flipping, stirring, serving. It washes easily, and it is thin enough to sever an unwieldy piece of chicken or zucchini should the need arise. But what I like the most is its scraping ability. With the leading edge flat against the #10 cast iron pan, I can salvage any crispies that may be stuck, be it potatoes or fried eggs. I turn the spatula over and repeat. Used in this manner, I imagine the metal becoming sharper with each pass across the black iron surface. Perhaps it will someday render my paring knife redundant.

The chainmail scrubber is used for cleaning said cast iron skillet. I rarely have respect for a kitchen tool that serves a single purpose, but for this, I make an exception. First of all, it is chainmail, real chainmail: interlocking rings that, in shirt form, protected both medieval knights and my Dungeons & Dragons characters from mortal injury, and that's just cool. The scrubber is not very big, just four inches square, but it's enough to do its job. All you need to do is add some warm water to the pan and scrub away. Bacon grease and elbow grease merge with the sound of metal grinding against metal, and the pan comes clean in less than 30 seconds. It is all so very satisfying. No soap is required. Then I give the pan a rinse and dry it right away with the designated dish towel (a permanently stained one). At the end of the day, the chainmail scrubber goes into the dishwasher.

And then there is the wooden spoon. Wood, that magical substance that people have been using for a few millennia. It never goes out of style. Joan of Arc, Billy the Kid, Genghis Khan, Abraham Lincoln, Socrates, and Bill & Ted—they all used wooden spoons. When you use a wooden spoon, you are one with history. I prefer a right-handed spoon, which has a nifty little angle to effectively scoop the bottom corner of the pot.

Hmmm . . . come to think of it, a few other "can't be without" kitchen items come to mind. There is the two-tined pot fork—13 inches long, very pointy. Unadulterated, culinary awesomeness. And the strainer! I use it for rinsing rice, getting the last drops of juice from orange pulp, and removing that gunk at the bottom of the cider vinegar bottle. I also can't forget the wide-mouthed canning funnel, which is utilized almost daily to fill thermoses with pasta or beans and rice for my daughters' lunches. Why do I hold this seemingly mundane tool in such high regard? It prevents drips, and in my world, kitchen counter drip prevention is one of the keys to marital harmony.

Okay, so that's seven items, I can count. Excuse me while I go stitch a few more holsters onto my utility belt.

He Who Smelt It

My daughter and I popped into a new fish store in Chico that advertised fresh-caught seafood. This is a pretty impressive statement for a business located nearly 200 road miles from the nearest coastal harbor. I asked my daughter what she thought would be good, and after surveying the offerings on the other side of the plexiglass, she eventually pointed to the smelt. Many people are squeamish when it comes to smelt. Too small to fillet, the six-inch-long fish are sold whole and are generally prepared breaded and fried. I was impressed with both the boldness of my daughter's choice, as well as the fact that these fish were from Half Moon Bay, which is about as locally-sourced an ocean fish as you can get if you live in Chico. We bought two pounds, which was probably close to 40 fish.

But how to cook them? I had a Red Lobster/Outback Steakhouse epiphany and thought of coconut shrimp. This seemed to me a logical connection; after all, the fish were roughly the same size as jumbo prawns, also came from the ocean, and we had some coconut flour in the pantry. It was all coming together perfectly! I imagined how the platter would look, with crispy, honey-colored delicacies laid out side-by-side in precise formation; the kitchen subtly filled with the combined scents of fresh seafood, coconut, and a dash of dried lemon thyme for a bit of mystique.

Two minutes after the fish hit the frying pan, I knew I was in trouble. Tails, heads, and middles were cooking at different rates. I tried to remedy the situation with my preferred kitchen weapon of choice—the spatula—but this just seemed to make things worse. My manipulations caused some fish to jackknife while others simply fell apart, disintegrating like lumps of sand in a rainstorm. The smelt refused to be flipped, and instead responded to my spatula as if it was a bulldozer, pushing miniature fish parts across the flat metal landscape as bits of spine and fin jutted out at odd angles.

Forget the serving platter. I reached for a large bowl into which I deposited the debris, placed caution tape around the pan, added more oil, and soldiered on to cook the remaining two dozen fish.

Reader take note: Coconut flour cooked with fish smells like fishy coconut (even with a dash of lemon thyme).

After opening the all the windows in the house, I nervously presented to my family a plate with four mostly honey-colored fish, neatly parallel-parked, and garnished with a bit of droopy kale.

"Didn't you buy two pounds?" asked my wife tentatively.

I sheepishly revealed the bowl, the contents of which resembled the greasy waste product from a cat-food factory. I served the intact fish to my wife and daughters, and then I tapped into my inner Dr. Frankenstein and carefully chose contents from the bowl to reassemble three more fish for myself. I could only manage to eat two of them. The third I tried to offer to the dog, who respectfully declined.

As I began to take out ingredients for hamburgers, the sunny voice of my four-year-old cut across the carnage of my culinary battlefield.

"More smelt, please!"

Dishwasher Safe?

It was my wife's favorite bowl. Earthy blue-grey, crafted by a college friend, the perfect size for a generous serving of rice and toppings. On this particular day, it carried a garden salad with greens and freshly-picked snap peas and some flower petals. My younger daughter held the bowl triumphantly in her hands, with my older daughter supporting her sister piggyback style. Until she stumbled. The bowl fell and broke into a dozen pieces. The peas were salvageable; the bowl was not. Our girls felt awful and promised to replace it, which they did. A few weeks later we were at an arts and crafts fair just before Mother's Day. One potter had a number of beautiful pieces for sale, all of which were out of my daughters' allowance budget. The sisters shared with him the story of how they had broken their mother's favorite bowl, and, moved by the sad tale as told by a nine- and a six-year-old, he gave them a bowl at a special reduced price of $1.

It is a beautiful piece of ceramic, the same size as its predecessor, blue, etched with images reminiscent of the flute-playing Kokopelli. It gets washed by hand, every day, sometimes more than once. Why? Because we never learned if it is dishwasher safe. Gabe, you inscribed your name on the bottom of the bowl, so if you read this, please let me know. Also, can we commission a couple more?

What's in the Soup?

Everything is in the soup. The drippings from last night's pork roast (or chicken, or beef, or lamb) form the base. If there are bones, toss them in too, but then add a splash of cider vinegar, to help dissolve some of the goodness. Throw in the pale bottom of the celery stalks or the parsley stems that no one wants to eat. Onion greens, garlic tops, borage from the back yard. Trimmings from radishes and turnips and beets and asparagus. Diced kale stems or cabbage stems or cauliflower stems or broccoli stems, a couple bay leaves from the tree by the creek, 10 peppercorns, some salt. Lamb's quarters and dandelion leaves—for weedy nutritious wildness. Herbs, whatever is on hand: whole sprigs of thyme, oregano, or rosemary. Lastly, a dash of cayenne to keep away the sniffles.

Fill the pot with water until the veggies are covered, bring to a boil. Let it simmer all day. Strain into a bowl, pour into quart jars and allow to cool. Squeeze the solids to get every last drop. At our house, the mush that remains goes to our chickens, which dutifully transform it into the next day's eggs. Two quarts of the broth go into the fridge, the rest to the freezer, to save for the next time a family member needs a mug of everything.

December Tomatoes

Initially saddened by the two dozen or so tomatoes that autumn had left green on the vine, I perked up when a friend explained to me a method by which those fruits could still achieve hues of ripeness. Before the first big frost of the fall (around the time you notice that those green tomatoes just aren't going to turn), pick any remaining green fruits and dump them into a paper bag. Add a whole, unripe banana. Place the bag in a cupboard, wait a week or two, and then, like magic, you have bona fide, ripe tomatoes.

It was too simple not to try. Just before the holidays, I pulled some tomatoes out of the cupboard—they looked ripe. . .ish. Kind of a pasty red. Not surprisingly, they were almost entirely devoid of flavor, and their texture was rather mealy. Now I know why recipes for fried green tomatoes exist.

Bitter Beets

Even butter can't make bitter beets taste better.

Arugula Pesto

I stopped planting arugula a number of years ago. There's just no sport in it. Sowing a bed of arugula is the gardening version of shooting fish in a barrel: it grows in any season, the slugs won't touch it, it reseeds itself, and isn't picky about how much water it gets. And seriously, there is a limit to the number of salads a person can make from this spicy green.

And yet, one December morning a stroll through the yard revealed not one, but two young thriving stands of the stuff. One patch had been seeded by my four-year-old, who had gone on a semi-supervised sowing binge a couple months prior. The clump of greens was growing rapidly and was slowly suffocating my feeble attempt at planting bok choy as well as encroaching upon ten diminutive caterpillar-ridden tatsoi plants. The second bunch of arugula had taken up residence a few feet away, emerging from wood chips next to a rose bush. How it got there I do not know, though I am thinking that the slugs planted it as a sick joke. The succession of mild winter days that followed proved to be perfect growing conditions for leafy greens. Three weeks later I found myself staring at a veritable hedgerow of arugula.

Someone once classified this spicy member of the mustard family as "food," so I felt obligated to make one final attempt to find some good recipes. I put together a diced tomato, onion, and arugula salsa-like mixture that was suggested as a topper for grilled salmon. It was delicious, but sadly it barely made a dent in the arugula supply. Even worse, the dark green jungle of leaves seemed to grow back minutes after being picked; within a day, there wasn't any evidence that my harvesting scissors had ever been there. I added some arugula to a batch of soup stock, but broth is something I only make a couple of times during the winter—far too infrequently for this particular need. The leaves provided a nice zip, but I was wary of the flavor becoming too overwhelming. Doing a select thinning of the arugula forest wasn't going to do it—I needed a recipe that called for a full-on clear-cut. But unlike tomatoes or zucchini, I really couldn't find many good options that used these mustardy greens en masse. The *Ball Jar Cookbook* doesn't have a listing for "arugula preserves," nor have I seen anyone trying pickled arugula ("Break out the canning jars, Hon. It's time to put up some rocket to get us through the hot, dry summer!").

I was finally led back to an arugula pesto recipe that had been suggested to me a few years ago. It called for swapping basil with arugula. Then I replaced pine nuts with farmers' market walnuts and tossed in some nutritional yeast as a substitute for grated Parmesan cheese (did I mention we are also mostly dairy-free?). I can't say it was a bad creation—perhaps a 7 or an 8 out of 10—but homemade pesto is supposed to be bowl-licking-delicious. It wasn't long before I placed the quart and a half of product in the freezer, where it played ugly stepsister to its roommates, three frozen logs of basil pesto leftover from the summer. By the time I ran out of the traditional pesto, I had only a couple months to wait before fresh basil started making an appearance again at the market. After consulting my taste buds, the decision was unanimous. The arugula pesto was filed away into the compost bin.

Just Grind It

One weekend, I was checking out one of the local antique stores and was amazed at the ingenuity of household appliances that existed before the invention of modern batteries or wall outlets. I was focusing especially on kitchen items with gears and cranks and handles, made of cast iron and wood and glass, and no electrical cords. These were gizmos that were built to last, and if broken, built to be diagnosed and fixed easily.

A food grinder caught my eye, and at just seven dollars, I couldn't resist. It was the type that clamps on to a counter and has various attachments, including one for making nut butter. I had been keen on locating one of these for a while, but was waiting to find one in good condition. Almonds are plentiful in our area, but good almond butter can be pricey. I knew that it wouldn't be long before the grinder paid for itself. Unfortunately, I was soon to learn that the "Just Grind It" attitude doth not almond butter make.

First, I roasted some almonds in the oven for about 20 minutes at about 200F degrees. I inserted a handful of nuts in the grinder and cranked. Or at least, I tried to. The clamp mechanism on the grinder didn't attach very well to any of my kitchen's surfaces, and it kept slipping. I eventually succeeded in securing it to the desk in the adjacent room with a couple of pieces of cardboard to protect the wood.

My second attempt was still hard work, and the grinder continued to slip. I did get some product though, but it was more of an almond meal consistency rather than a butter. I put the almonds back in the oven to roast for another 15 minutes, this time at 300F degrees.

The third attempt produced similar results with similar effort, though perhaps the consistency was slightly more creamy. That's what I told myself, anyway—denial is strong in this one. My final effort involved pre-chopping the almonds. Grinding became a bit easier, but the results didn't change. Perhaps I didn't have the right variety of almonds. To add insult to injury, cleaning the grinder after use was no small chore.

The silver lining is that the almond meal goes well in waffle batter and adds a nice flavor to yogurt. There are also other attachments for the grinder, so if I want to, I can experiment with demolishing other foods. For the time being, I'm putting this endeavor into the "Well, I tried" category. There must be something to this apparently complicated culinary art that I am missing.

Success

A common recommendation made by doctors is to eat healthy amounts of yogurt after completing a course of antibiotics. The idea here is that healthy bacteria in the yogurt will help give the "good" bacteria in your digestive tract a boost, as the antibiotic caused these beneficial critters to suffer the same fate as the "bad" bacteria.

Of course, the practice of eating foods with live, active cultures predates both Western medical advice as well as the latest "raw, fermented" fad by quite a few centuries. Yogurt is a classic example, as are kimchi, miso, cheese, and dozens of other culinary favorites. Not wanting my family to miss out on the latest health craze, I purchased a 16-ounce jar of raw, naturally-fermented sauerkraut. While I was doubtful everyone would enjoy it, my wife and I did our best to set the stage. "Try this—it tastes like pickles." Our elder daughter was wary, but she was a good sport and took a spoonful. Then she wanted seconds. And thirds. What about our one-year-old? Would lightning strike twice? The answer was a resounding "yes," and soon she, too, was putting her fingers together, giving us the baby-sign for "more."

I read up on sauerkraut. It seemed to be extremely simple to make. All you need to do is shred a cabbage, add a bit of salt, and set the mixture aside in an out-of-the-way place for a couple of weeks. I did the math: the price tag on a 16-ounce jar of raw organic artisan sauerkraut is $8.79. Local cabbage goes for $1/lb. By simply letting the cabbage spoil, its value increases by a factor of almost 20! It was too good to be true, and I had to try it.

However, after failed attempts at fabricating my own almond butter, kale chips, and peach jam (I ended up having to call it syrup), I must admit that I entered into this project with a certain sense of trepidation. Even a couple of DIY friends who make their own yummy gourmet porridge out of native grass seed and field weeds told me that they only had about a 20% success rate with making sauerkraut. But I figured the worst thing that could happen would be creating a stinking culture of deadly poisonous bacteria in the kitchen. So I bought two cabbages from my local farmer and started chopping.

The key to sauerkraut is making sure the good bacteria—which naturally exist on the cabbage—are "happy" and that everything else, including airborne molds, insects, and other bacteria, have no access to the cabbage. This requires a certain appreciation for keeping things clean—ideally sterile—and this, in turn, requires patience, which is yet another perpetual challenge for some of us.

Complicating matters were conflicting strategies on how to make the sauerkraut. The most common instructions call for a dinner plate and a mixing bowl, where the plate just fits inside the top of the bowl. Shredded cabbage and salt go into the bowl, the plate goes on the cabbage, and a weight (like a smaller bowl filled with water) goes on the plate. My problem was that I shredded the cabbage first and then started looking for the right sized plate and bowl. However, the clock was ticking: once you mix the cabbage and salt, you cover it with a towel and then let it sit for up to 45 minutes before transferring it to the bowl where it will ferment. What happens after 45 minutes? I wasn't sure, but I didn't want my house to become the first spoiled cabbage Superfund site. There was no time to waste.

It took me 10 minutes to find a couple of possible bowl-plate options. In went the shredded cabbage, on went the plate. But the plate didn't fit; there was too much cabbage. Take two. I transferred the cabbage to a bigger bowl, put my plate on, but this time there was a gap of air between the plate and the cabbage. This was a no-no. So I put the cabbage back into the first bowl and squished down as hard as I could. No dice. I just had too much material.

Common sense would dictate removing some of the cabbage, but it had taken me over a half hour just to chop the stuff, and I had no desire to compost a quarter of it for want of a correctly-sized container. Nor did I want to attempt two batches, which would only double my chance of failure. So back to the computer I went.

A couple of websites suggested using a plastic Ziploc bag filled with water to take the place of both the plate and the weight. Instead of a bowl, the directions called for a large glass jar. Once the jar is stuffed about ¾ of the way with cabbage, the bag of water fills the remaining space, and keeps air away from the mixture.

But by now my 45-minute time limit had expired. Panic set in, as I imagined that the contamination of my fledgling experiment had already begun. Desperate times call for desperate measures. I put the entire mess into the pasta colander and rinsed, hopefully flushing all of the invisible (or imagined) bacterial nasties down the drain. I put the sopping cabbage back in the mixing bowl, added more salt, and then followed the rest of the instructions. By the time I placed my mixture in the cupboard, the entire kitchen, along with much of my body, looked like the aftermath of a ticker-tape parade of damp cabbage shavings. It took another 40 minutes to restore order, and it was well after midnight before I got to bed.

Over the next week, the contents of the jar turned from a light green to a dull yellow. I watched carefully for mysterious molds and sniffed daily for foul non-krauty aromas. I remained vigilant for signs of contamination, including fuzz, orange spots, and dead canaries but noted nothing out of the ordinary. After twelve days, it was time.

It is bad luck to be superstitious, but I crossed my fingers anyway as I pulled out the plastic bag. With a damp cloth I wiped the rim and upper part of the inside of the jar, and as a precaution, carefully spooned out the top half inch of sauerkraut and placed it in the compost bin.

I sampled some. It was tangy, salty, cabbagy, and satisfyingly crunchy. Miraculously, it seemed, well, perfect. My wife tried a spoonful and she concurred that it was delicious. Our daughters wanted to try some. They loved it. Twenty-four hours passed and no emergency room visits were necessary. Two weeks later, I repeated my success. And then I did it again, this time adding some shaved carrots. And then again, with chunks of daikon radish.

I am the King of Kraut, and my family loves me for it.

Sour Grapes and Dour Gripes
(a.k.a Things I Really Don't Like)

☹ Straws. I hate straws. Single-use plastic straws are just gratuitous pointless waste. I even think compostable paper straws are silly. I mean, unless you are genuinely requiring a straw for medical reasons, who really needs a factory to turn tree pulp into a paper straw? Have we really forgotten how to drink beverages directly with our lips? ("Oh, but that straw in the plastic lid makes it so much more convenient, and it helps prevent spills!"). I call B.S. I have seen plenty of spills from lidded cups sporting straws. Perhaps the next worse thing to disposable straws are "ecofriendly" reusable straws—metal, plastic or bamboo (yes, I have also seen those). My kids love them, but they are not designed for the dishwasher, and I can think of a thousand things I would rather do with my time than hand-clean a straw with a soap-covered pipe cleaner.

☹ Items that you can recycle or compost in some cities, but not most cities, and certainly not my city, like aseptic packaging (a.k.a. Tetra paks). Or items that tout they come in biodegradable plastic containers, which really only biodegrade if your community has an industrial composting facility, which again, mine does not.

☹ Who the hell thought it was necessary to reinvent the water bottle? My message to you: More complicated is not better. Too many of today's water bottles are intricate to the point that they trigger Muphy's Law. They have complicated flip-top lids, internal straws, and removable washers, all of which beg to get broken or lost. Both outcomes occur frequently with my family. My wife even bought a special stainless steel pry-tool for removing the washers. (Perhaps this is more sanitary than a paperclip or small flathead screwdriver.)

Two brushes can be purchased to clean the bottle, one for the straws and another for the bottle itself. And clean you must, as it is easy for gunk to accumulate around every small hinge and crevice. Forget running the bottle through the dishwasher—it is "double-wall insulated," which translates to "hand wash only or your dishwasher will blow up."

Back in the day, when we wanted to keep our water cold, we added (drum roll please) . . . ICE CUBES. Nor do all these extra "conveniences" make these water bottle leak-proof or spill-proof. Trust me, I have experience in these matters. When did people abandon their appreciation for the utilitarian wide-mouth Nalgene? Or the spaceship shaped boy scout canteen? Or the bota bag?

☹ Sticker labels on individual apples, bananas, and avocados. Is this really necessary?

☺ Slugs, earwigs, leaf-footed bugs, spiders that catch bees instead of mosquitoes . . .

☹ Gas-powered leaf blowers: loud, toxic, and unnecessary.

Okay, I think that's enough dour for now.

Verse and Versatility

Potluck

Todd's a meat fanatic, he won't touch salad greens
    The Smiths are vegan folk, and forgo steak and spleen.
Abby avoids all cheese, she says it gives her gas
    And if Eric eats a tree nut, that bite will be his last.
I offer Leah shrimp kabob, she says, politely, "No sir"
    And then I am reminded—crustaceans are not kosher.
Chris says garlic's off the table, Tom is gluten free
    Megan avoids all Oscar Meyer (which is quite fine with me).
Amy goes against the grains; she says it's better for her system.
    "Would you like to know the ingredients, Dear?"
    "Yes, please. Go ahead and list 'em"
Duke don't dance with pineapple juice, Nikki doesn't drink
    Sam shuns added sucrose, and the nightshades too, I think.
In the end we all sat at the table, and I guess the time was nice.
    We swapped stories and clinked glasses;
    we dined on water with no ice.

Ode to Kale Stems

The employee at Sweetgreens in Rockefeller Center
    was shucking the leaves off the dino kale,
    discarding the stems.
The kale was from California, according to the box
The same kale I purchase at the local store
    when I cannot get to the farmers' market
    or when it is out of season, and I have a need for greens.

I could use those stems.
I would dice them with onion, and mix them into meatballs
I would chop them into a bean salad
I would sneak them into potato pancakes
I would add them to soup
I would feed them to the chickens

I want to claim them before they become green waste,
    but they won't fit in my carry-on
And I am 2,500 miles from my home.

Grandma's Cuisinart

The Cuisinart belonged to my grandmother-in-law
Used for decades to prep latkes or 'slaw
Or slice cucumbers quickly
Always patched, never broken, the blade still whirs with the ferocity of a tiger who craves chopped nuts.
Keep your hand pressed firmly on the lid, lest the contents erupt like Lassen back in '15
The most important joints are now made of epoxy.
I say this with moxy.
as I blend gazpacho.

Dear Chef Gezunt[1]

Dear Chef Gezunt,

I am very disappointed with twist ties these days. They just aren't what they used to be. I recall twist ties that were plastic, strong, and could secure a produce bag like Fort Knox. Now all I see are these wimpy, paper-covered wires. I might as well just tie my bags shut with a knot, and then open them back up with a steak knife. Do quality twist ties still exist?

~ Seeking Closure in Corning

Dear Seeking Closure,

Truly, I feel your pain. Fortunately, I know where you can find the twist tie you desire. Look no further than a package of coffee. Many coffee packages are designed to be recloseable by way of the most awesome twist ties ever created—a plastic strap, ¼" wide and up to 7" long, made flexible by twin parallel wires embedded within. I find them to be quite reusable, and as durable as industrial-strength zip-ties. When I finish a package of coffee, I remove the closure piece and set it aside in the utility drawer. I have used them for everything from hanging tools in my garage to securing a wire basket on the back of a bike. As far as the paper-covered wire ties that you find in the produce section, I find that twisting two of them together (like a two-stranded cord) increases both their durability and longevity.

Dear Chef Gezunt,

What is the most versatile non-food item in your kitchen?

~Pocketknife Patti in Paradise

Dear Pocketknife Patti,

That's a fine question. I would have to say that the glass jar is the winner of my versatility award. When many people think of jars, they think of fruit and vegetable preserves—perhaps a batch of salsa, or

---

1. Chef Gezunt is not a professional chef, nor does he play one on Netflix or Hulu. But he is a real person.

storing summer's peach bounty for a sweet January treat. But for my family, this is just the tip of the iceberg. Watertight and microwave safe, glass jars are used to hold everything from dried herbs to frozen chicken broth to leftover ratatouille. I keep a 4-oz jar in the fridge stocked with peeled garlic cloves, while large quart jars in the pantry hold Moroccan spice mix, dry beans, and rice. We have special screw-on lids with a pour spout feature which enable us to turn wide mouth jars into pitchers for orange juice or coffee. When wrapped with a bow, jars make great gift vessels for holiday granola, roasted nuts or soup mixes. Jars can also serve as drinking glasses, vases, or, in a pinch, rolling pins. Not bad for something that was invented in 1803. All this for an item that is inexpensive, non-toxic, dishwasher safe, and fully recyclable.

Dear Chef Gezunt,

I cook a lot of food in the oven, and my broiler drip tray can get pretty gross with slimy, greasy gunk. I recall my mom dumping the drippings down the drain, but I am concerned about clogs. Perhaps I can save the gunk and mix it in with the dog food? What are your thoughts on this?

~ Drip Tray Trey in Gridley

Dear Drip Tray Trey,

Don't dump those drippings! There are chefs that consider those juices to be gastronomic gold (provided that they aren't burned). In my book, they are what is known in the culinary world as a "reduction," where the flavor of a liquid mixture (such as a soup or sauce) is made more intense by simmering or boiling. When the liquid in the drip tray is still warm, I carefully pour it through a fine (or sometimes coarse) wire-mesh sieve into an appropriate-sized glass jar. Then I loosely screw on a lid and set it aside to cool. The solids left behind in the sieve—which might include peppercorns, herb stems, and the like—can be composted (or fed to chickens). Depending on what you cooked, there may be a layer of fat the rises to the top of the liquid, and, if put in the fridge, this will eventually solidify. If you wish, you can separate the two once the jar cools. I often use the fat (pork fat =

lard, beef fat = tallow, poultry fat = schmaltz) in savory dishes in place of butter or olive oil. Meanwhile, the tasty, high-nutrient liquid has several applications, including as a soup base or as a flavoring for rice or cooked vegetable dishes. (And while we are on the topic of soups, feel free to toss in some of the vinegary liquid from a jar of olives or dill pickles. Both will add flavor as well as aid in helping to dissolve soup bones, which further boosts the nutritional value of your broth.) The drippings store well in the freezer, but keep the lids screwed on loosely until the liquid freezes lest you risk cracking the glass jar. I would not recommend using it as pet food, however, as the high fat content may not be healthy for your furry friend.

Dear Chef Gezunt,

I want to take a break from my processed food snacks—trail mix bars and the occasional cookie have been my go-to's. Can you recommend a good, simple, tasty replacement that doesn't come in a package?

~Noshy Nancy in Chico

Dear Noshy Nancy,

I'm glad you asked! My current favorite snack starts with a crisp apple. I slice it in half and remove the core with a pointed paring knife. Then I spread roughly a tablespoon of plain peanut or almond butter on each half and sprinkle with salt. It's a great mid-morning pick-me-up or lunchtime dessert.

CHAPTER 2

In Search of the Green Thumb

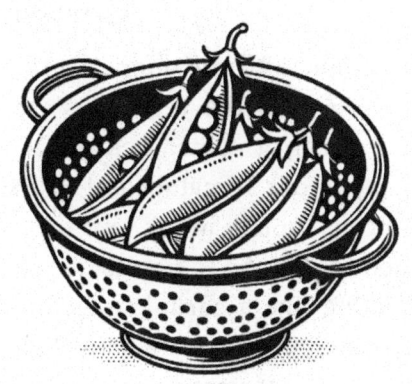

Tarzan the Gardener

My bookshelf includes treatises on organic gardening, permaculture, companion planting, and compost care, but this is mostly to delude myself into thinking that I am some sort of god-figure in my garden with the power to repel aphids, make peaches ripen on command, and lower the pH of my soil with a single flick of my trowel. While I don't have the ability to do these things, I have browsed every page of my gardening books as if they were Hogwarts textbooks containing spells to ward off cabbage worms or grow the sweetest peppers. Some of these pages I have even marked with Post-Its, but that really doesn't mean much. I get advice from friends and farmers about tomato watering and snail abatement strategies, but my mind is like a well-drained soil—some concepts are absorbed, but there is much that just percolates through. I try to weed out the ideas that don't work and save the seeds of the ones that do, but somehow it all seems to end up jumbled in the compost heap of gardening wisdom. I even have grandiose visions of keeping a gardening journal from year to year and of mapping where each plant will reside. But a bigger part of me desires to embrace the simplicity of a "Tarzan the Farmer" mentality: "Dig! Plant seed! Water! Grow! Eat!" Somewhere in between diligence and naivety, my garden turns into a jungle, and Tarzan is happy. And the gophers are happy. And the snails. And the weeds. And the zucchini.

Companion Planting

The topic of companion planting comes up again and again. These days, I guess even the vegetables are pressured to find a soul partner. Does that mean a solitary carrot is incomplete without its romaine lettuce companion? Tomatoes and basil seem to be the most frequently mentioned pairing, though in my yard they appear far from being bosom buddies. In fact, I think the tomatoes have unfriended the basil entirely, leaving them looking like a shrunken-leafed, twiggy, Mojave Desert version of basil rather than a specimen worthy of a fragrant herbal bouquet one might find at the farmers' market. Where I have basil growing in full sun, the plants seemed to have gone from being newly emerged sprouts to sending up seedy flower heads over a couple of weeks. Meanwhile, the more shaded plants still have just a single pair of leaves, two months into the summer. By the end of the season, I should have just enough basil to make a couple teaspoons of pesto.

Garden Sisters

The widely acclaimed "Three Sisters" garden is the holy grail of companion planting. It is a utopian integration of beans, corn, and winter squash that was planted, in various forms, by Native peoples throughout much of North America. In a nutshell, here is how it is supposed to work: the corn (usually a "dent" corn with kernels that are ground into a flour) is planted first followed a few weeks later by a vining variety of bean and a winter squash such as pumpkin or butternut. Symbiotic bacteria on the roots of the beans free up nitrogen in the soil, which improves the growth and yield of the corn and squash. The corn provides a living pole for the beans to climb. Meanwhile, as the squash vines spread out below, their large leaves impede weed growth and reduce the evaporation of moisture from the soil. In some regions, sunflowers are included as a "fourth sister" to aid in pollination by attracting bees.

This is all fine and good if the sisters get along, and I would guess the Native Americans were able to establish rules of the house to enforce horticultural harmony. Unfortunately, I didn't remember to bookmark the page describing how to encourage the sisters to play nice together, so much of what my yard experiences is sibling rivalry.

It started with the beans, which the previous season were so vigorous that they all but collapsed the corn, so the following year I separated them by alternating rows of corn with bean towers. The corn has decided to pout by producing a single ear for every five stalks. Once the corn worms take their share, each ear has about ten kernels left, enough for a couple of bites, except when my daughter gets impatient and plucks an ear too early (though at two years old, each bite for me is equivalent to five for her). Meanwhile, the beans flaunt their success by producing pods faster than I can pick them. The squash, on the other hand, struggles to grow in the shade of its taller sisters.

Towering over all this activity like gentle giants are three sunflower plants, which have topped out at about 11 feet. The sunflowers reseed each year and have gracefully established themselves as the peacemakers among their sisters: they tolerate the embrace of the bean vines and watch over the corn, squash, and the rest of the garden with a warmth of summer that only sunflowers can emanate. Spiders, beetles, aphids, praying mantis, caterpillars, and multiple species of bees and wasps all pay their respect to the sunflowers during these months; come fall, birds will dine on the seeds, and in the process will scatter a few for next year. The sunflowers are the true queens of the garden landscape. They are the first plant that catches my eye in the morning, and their thick stalks and dried flower heads remain as sentinels in the yard long after the November frosts put an inevitable end to the summer bounty. Friends ask me how I managed to get them to grow so well. I answer that I had little to do with it. And that is how it should be.

Tomato Envy

I go over to a friend's garden in late June to discover rambunctious 7-foot tall plants neatly tied to a row of six 8-foot high trellises. Firm green fruits are scattered among a galaxy of yellow flowers, and a handful of tomatoes are already ripening at the base of the tower—all this despite record low temperatures over the previous month. Meanwhile, I think of my own diminutive garden-gnome sized plants that are struggling to send out flowers, most of which are withering and dying without setting fruit. I am consumed with tomato envy.

Of course, I have only myself to blame. That, and the culture of tomato snobbery that has infected our society and brainwashed me into believing that any plant not labeled "heirloom" may be fine enough for the peasants who buy their tomato starts from the big-box hardware store, but I am a connoisseur and above such low-brow cultivating. Yes, "Ace," "Early Girl" and "Better Boy" are all perfectly fine brand-name hybrid tomatoes, but the heirlooms, well, you know, they sound so cool. I mean, who wouldn't want to plant the "Cosmonaut Volkov," or "Black from Tula, or "Earl of Edgecombe"? But perhaps I have lost track of the real goal, which is to actually produce something to eat. I ponder this possibility as I reminisce on last-year's "Brandywine, Sudduth Strain" harvest, a single fruit that I impatiently plucked too early.

No, no, please don't offer me any advice at this point. I want to hear none of those witch doctor ideas about pruning the tomato vines, or precision-timed watering schedules, or applying Epsom salts, or how to inject earthworm castings into the soil in April and again in July. Tarzan the Gardener would never do such things.

But here is what I will do. I will go out and plant 19 different tomato plants with 18 different names. Of these, nine will be from the farmers' market. Two will have been started by 4th graders, purchased at a local school fundraiser. Three will be "rescue plants" from the neighbor who started 60 plants in her mini-greenhouse and only has room in her yard for six. Four will be plants that I started from seed in the windowsill that managed to survive the slugageddon incident of April 2011 (I began with two dozen). And the last one—the healthiest of all—will suddenly appear between two butternut squash plants, having sprouted from a seed that had been patiently lying dormant in soil at the bottom of the compost bin, just waiting for its moment.

Some will be planted in the shadow of a lavender thicket that hums with honeybees, and others will be shaded for three hours a day by a 100-foot redwood. Some will get moisture every time I spray down the adjacent cucumber plants, a handful will be on the same underground soaker hose line that is irrigating the summer squash, and a few will get a couple gallons of water every now and again just when I feel like it. All will be planted up to two feet deep in some of the finest alluvial soil the Sacramento Valley has to offer. Most of them will be heirlooms, and the hope is, that when all is said and done, there will be enough tomatoes to make my family happy. I am sure some will do well, and some will not, but here is my theory: while I am far too lazy to actually follow through on any sound advice I have been given about how to grow a particular heirloom variety, I do know that there are about 3,000 cultivars of heirloom tomatoes presently being grown on the planet, each one specifically bred for a certain soil, climate, or culinary purpose. All I need to do is figure out which one is best adapted for my style of gardening and hope that it has a really cool name. Or I can go purchase a few discounted "Better Boys" from Lowe's.

Mystery Mix

As I was helping to clean up at the conclusion of an annual Seed Swap, I noted that one of the folding tables was sprinkled with loose seeds of all shapes and sizes. These were the casualties from seed swappers who were too hasty in transferring their garden dreams from cryptically labeled jars into small wax paper bags, or perhaps the seeds were escapees from poorly-made seed packets with openings at both ends. I used my hand to make a small hill of seeds on the corner of the table, and then carefully pushed them over the edge into an envelope which I labeled "Mystery Mix." These couple of hundred seeds joyfully found their way into a three-square-foot section of my daughter's garden bed, where a couple months later, they exploded into a raucous bouquet of watermelon, poppies, cherry tomatoes, beans, morning glory, and more. At the end of the season, I cleared the frosty, brown crinkly thicket of shrubbery and found a small but healthy celery plant growing in the protection of the expired vines and musty leaves. It was the first time I had ever seen celery growing in my yard, ever.

Observations I

 A morning walk reveals an unexpected flash of purple in the joint of the sidewalk. A pansy, also known as a Johnny Jump Up, simply happy to be growing amidst the sea of concrete. Around the corner, a different color. An emerald green sweat bee, its metallic sheen dusted with pollen, scurries around a blue Bachelor's Button flower. Does it know how pretty it looks or how unique?

- Of all the roses in our yard, it is the native California rose (*Rosa californica*) that smells the sweetest, and once picked, is the first to drop its petals, as if to say, "Leave me in the wild and not in a vase on the countertop."

- When weeding, if you pull petty spurge up near the base of the plant, the sap is less likely to stain and chap your fingers. Of course, as my wife and daughters remind me, if I were to wear garden gloves, I wouldn't have to worry about the sap at all.

- My beans are spiraling up their poles in a counterclockwise manner. Apparently, all beans do this—spiral counterclockwise as they climb—regardless of whether you are in the Northern Hemisphere or the Southern Hemisphere. There is a gene that codes for it. Nobody seems to know why.

Garlic and Spuds[1]

My track record for gardening consistency is, sadly, mixed. I am not a rock star with tomatoes, or cucumbers, or even zucchini. But I do have a bread and butter: I figured out how to grow garlic and potatoes. Toss those two with olive oil, salt, and fresh rosemary and you're on your way to a side dish that pleases everyone.

Here's how I do it: first, you make sure that gophers can't get into your garden boxes. This actually took me a few years, with the final step being removing all of the soil from the garden box, re-lining the bottom and the sides of the eight-year-old cedar-wood frame with wire mesh, and then shoveling the soil back in.

From there it's easy-peasy, my favorite type of gardening. First and foremost, there are no seeds to plant, so I never have to be concerned about failed germination. For the garlic, I keep track of when the garlic heads from the farmers' market start sprouting green stems, usually in December. I carefully separate the sprouting cloves and plant them four to six inches apart, stem oriented upwards, about an inch deep in the damp

---

[1]. I extend my gratitude to Lee and Francine at GRUB Farm for their sound advice regarding the cultivation and storage of potatoes and garlic.

winter soil. Within two weeks the stems can be seen emerging through the winter frost. I start watering once the earth begins to dry out in the early spring, and by April, the garlic heads are plump enough to gather as needed, a couple of plants at a time. The leaves are also flavorful in soups. The final harvest takes place in June once the leaves start to dry out. I hang them in bunches of six or so for three weeks to ensure the leaves dry completely, after which I store them, ideally away from the summer heat. I tried braiding the dried stems once, but this requires skill (which I lack) and garlic plants of uniform size (which I never have). I usually have enough garlic left over to plant again the following winter.

The process for potatoes is similar. In February, I set aside some smaller farmers' market potatoes and wait for the "eyes" to start bulging with little white or pink bumps, depending on the variety of spud. In mid-March (some suggest St. Patrick's Day), I dig fist-deep holes in loose soil about a foot apart and lob a single potato into each. Then I fill the holes and keep the soil moist. Depending on the soil temperature, the plants start emerging within 2-3 weeks, first forming a crack in the surface of the earth and then bursting out with small, green pom-poms of leaves over a matter of days. I have been informed that Father's Day is the time when you harvest potatoes, but I have dug up some small potatoes in late May, and I have left others in the ground through much of the summer. The real treat, of course, is waiting for a day when my daughters have some friends over, and then I suggest a potato hunt. There is a special joy in watching kids paw through the dirt seeking buried, edible treasures. We usually celebrate with a potato feast, flavored generously with garlic.

It Came from the Compost Bin

A squash plant sporting light-green orbs had thrust its way out of the pile of debris in the compost bin. The bin is an edifice constructed of four rickety wood pallets held together with scraps of rope and containing a mixture of dirt, pulled-up weeds, and yard trimmings that Mother Nature keeps at the perfect temperature for housing worms, centipedes, beetles, ants, lizards, pillbugs, earwigs, the occasional rat, and rogue squash plants. I have read that in order for the decomposition process to occur at its full potential, the temperature of the bin must be somewhere north of the ambient air temperature. The gold standard for a compost bin is one that is hot and steamy. Mine is always cold and clammy. There is a recipe for composting, and I tried to follow it, really I did. I added greens, browns, water, I turned it, massaged it, and fed it my choicest kitchen scraps. The internet tells of one guy that got his compost bin so hot that he used it to slow-cook his Thanksgiving turkey. My compost bin couldn't slow cook a salad.

Despite my failures, I do know this: over the course of the year, everything in the compost bin does become soil. Well, everything but the weed seeds (these turn into weeds). However, this does not keep me from extracting rich earth from the bottom of the bin for use in amending the nearby garden beds. While the compost bin conspires with my postage-stamp lawn to maintain a substantial herbarium of Northern California's weed varieties, the presence of a single, ginormous, healthy volunteer summer squash plant somehow turns every weed into an afterthought. Even as the basil languishes next to the tomatoes, the 3-foot-high, 6-foot-long zucchini plant snakes across the wood-chipped landscaping and onto the pathway, as if it is attempting to fulfill its lifelong dream of being a stunt double for a future sequel to *It's the Great Pumpkin, Charlie Brown*.

As summer progresses I realize that the romance of this situation could get out of hand. I ponder this as I grab my machete for another expedition to the yard. The nutrient-rich soil is a cradle not just for volunteer squash but also for a chaotic garden jungle. Cucumber vines are merging with the cherry tomato plants to form a twisted, mad-scientist "cucumato" bush. They are probably doing this to escape the substantial shadows cast by three large chard plants a few feet away, which themselves are the last holdouts from the winter garden. I resist yanking them out of admiration for their tenacity and ability to survive the full range of Chico's weather. Of course, now that the chard stalks are worthy of a logging operation, removing them at this point would leave substantial craters behind as well as pull up half the cucumber plants in their wake. So a couple times a month I take my knife to the chard leaves, cook up about 1/3 of the harvest, and store the rest in the fridge for a few more weeks until it is time to empty the mushy, forgotten remains onto the compost bin. The cucumber plants share no gratitude for my efforts, and as of August 1st, haven't yet produced a single fruit. Meanwhile, jealous of the zucchini, the watermelon vines are getting bored of the garden and are beginning to explore the lawn. But what did I spy popping up among the watermelon vines? Basil plants, as healthy as can be. I went on Facebook and it is true—the melons have added basil as a friend.

Eggplants of Winter

The seed fairy struck again, this time in late October, and this time with eggplant. Telling your preschooler that eggplant seeds are usually sown indoors in early March is just impolite. She asked where a good place to plant them would be, and I found an empty terracotta pot, which I placed outside next to our garden box. We added fresh compost and she carefully emptied the contents of the entire package, perhaps three dozen seeds, onto an area roughly the size of a dinner plate. We watered it occasionally, and as the night-time temperatures began to dip, I brought the pot inside into our sunroom off the kitchen. A meadow of weeds and miscellaneous kitchen-scrap sproutlings soon emerged (which we diligently removed), but a few days later young eggplant leaves peeked up over the lip of the pot, probably wondering what that hell they were doing growing two weeks before Thanksgiving. Over the next month I secretly thinned these down to six evenly spaced plants. We kept watering, and they kept growing.

Unfortunately, our sunroom only has south-facing windows, so the plants began to take on Wilt Chamberlain-type attributes as they elongated toward the low winter sun. The leaves became a pasty, anemic green, and I had to console the plants, reminding them that even though they might feel miserable—with their roots balled up in a pot in a room with only a little natural light—that outside, the morning temperatures were killing off avocado and citrus trees, and a poor eggplant wouldn't stand a chance.

They must have appreciated my kind words, for a few days later, the leggy stems pushed out pale lavender flowers. These would remain for a week at a time, and then turn tan and fall off. The whole scene was depressing. If my sunroom was a zoo, PETA advocates would be pounding at my door. I kept hoping to see an actual fruit, but this has the prerequisite of pollen moving from one flower to another. Unfortunately, this indoor space had no wind and no insects, and so there would be no fertilization. It was time to take matters into my own hands, literally.

Armed with a Q-tip, I generously budgeted four minutes of time to poking into one eggplant flower after another, twisting the cotton gently each time. While I tried to liken myself to a bee, the whole experience actually made me feel a bit uncomfortable. But it worked. A week later, two marble-sized eggplants appeared beneath the foliage. This being February in Northern California, these were probably the only eggplants growing for at least 200 miles in any direction.

After three weeks, one fruit had swelled to the grand size of—excuse the cliché—an egg. Its companion had shriveled. Upon closer inspection, the room was not devoid of insect life after all, as a fine, ivory netting was curling up the leaves of one of the plants, and was inhabited by a population of tiny white critters. Fearing that the days of edibility for the one eggplant were numbered, I harvested it, momentarily admired the mottled green and purple striping, and then sliced it and fried it in a bit of butter. It took 5 seconds to eat, with my wife, daughter, and I each getting a share.

A warming spell in mid-April signified it was time to get the garden started. The last frost date had passed. I looked in the sunroom: the eggplants, each about 20-inches tall, were still there and, somehow, still alive, albeit in a "Han Solo encased in carbonite" sort of way. They had survived the winter, and it was time to release them from their prison. We dug six generous holes in a garden bed and then dislodged the plants from the pot. The roots had almost completely replaced the compost and resembled a cylinder-shaped ball of twine. We separated the plants as best as we could and placed them in the holes. I later staked the wiry, pencil-thick stems, tying them gently.

As compared to the verdant eggplants starts that were beginning to appear at the local nurseries, these plants looked like zombies. The twiggy stalks had leaves like toy T-Rex arms and appeared just as pitiful. The cool soil was a shock to the plants, and over the next two days they looked like they were ready for hospice. The top six inches of the plants looked truly dead, and these I clipped. Still worried, I did the last thing I could think of. I bought four eggplant starts, which I planted in the adjacent garden bed.

It is May 3 as I type this, and the daytime temperatures have just begun to hit the low 90s. If you ever have a desire to tell a four-year-old that eggplants shouldn't be planted in October because they won't survive, don't. It just isn't true.

Dill and Cucumbers

Some of the tastiest dishes reflect the seasonality of their ingredients. A late summer garden consisting of tomatoes, eggplant, onions, zucchini, sweet peppers, and herbs can translate into delicious ratatouille. In the early winter, parallel rows of cabbage, beets, and potatoes can be the base for a filling borscht stew. It is even suggested that planting key ingredients side by side will improve the growth and flavor of both. Tomatoes and basil are the poster children for this technique.

Such were the images in my mind when in late April I planted dill adjacent to pickling cucumbers. Pop culture websites support such ventures, like this inspirational tidbit from the official-sounding "gardenguides.com":

> *Cucumbers and dill are meant to be together from garden row to pickle jar. Aromatic dill repels insect pests such as cucumber beetles that can decimate a cucumber crop.*

Seriously, how can you beat "meant to be together?" Denying two vegetables the opportunity for such a romance to blossom would be a tragedy of Shakespearean proportions.

Also, pickles are a favorite in my family. When all else fails, place a slice of pickle between two pieces of bread and my younger daughter is very happy. We planted seeds; the cucumber sprouts soon emerged, followed a week later by a delicate, green carpet of dill. And then I blinked. Before the cuke's had gained their second set of leaves, the dill had flowered and set seed. The plants had reached a height of five inches before a May heatwave nudged them to the next stage of their life cycle. (A pretty big let down for a seed variety named "Mammoth.)

It's just not fair.

In my area, it would be too cold to plant the dill any sooner. Plant it later, and the challenge (for me) becomes the watering requirements. I use a buried soaker hose in the summer to reduce evaporation; as a result, I don't have to water as frequently. My garden bed often appears dry even though there is plenty of moisture just below the surface. However, this is not agreeable for dill seeds, which are sown at just a quarter-inch deep and need to remain moist until the plants are well-established. Employing two different watering schemes for the same bed is more than I have the time or will to attempt. Besides, if one package of dill yields only enough material for half a pickle, then what's the point?

Perhaps other gardeners have better luck. (Actually, I am sure other gardeners have better luck). At least I gain some consolation from our local farmers' market, my personal barometer for measuring my gardening prowess/ineptitude, where I have yet to see pickling cucumbers and dill weed being sold on the same day.

The Volunteer

I added a new raised garden bed this winter in the following, unscientific, wing-it manner:

Step 1: Painstakingly line the bed with hardware cloth in an attempt to discourage gophers.

Step 2: Fill the bottom of the bed with random yard trimmings that you never want to see again (like thorny rose stems).

Step 3: Fill the remainder of the bed with two parts soil dug from random places in the yard and one part compost from the bottom of "ye ole" compost heap, complete with red worms, pill bugs, ants, centipedes, and a menagerie of partially-decomposed vegetable matter consisting of kitchen scraps and last year's garden foliage.

The neat part about this kind of raised bed construction is that it grows its own garden. Certainly I expected the soil and compost to be saturated with the seeds of borage, sunflowers, and the usual weedy suspects of petty spurge, groundsel, and prickly lettuce. But then there was also a tomato sprout, a small potato plant, the distinct spade-shaped leaves of a young bean, two squash seedlings, and a young walnut tree (which I yanked).

It is the squash that I watched most warily. With tomatoes or potatoes, you generally know what you are going to get, but with feral squash, it is a crapshoot whether or not the plant will produce fruit worthy of the dinner table. Years ago, I had an experience with a compost cucurbit that resulted in an oversized zucchini-like creature with flesh as tough as a tree root. I learned this the hard way when I tried to carve it for Halloween and ended up snapping the tip off of my kitchen knife. In the end I whittled and sawed at it as if it were a wood block, creating an evil Aliens-like monster that I mounted into the side of a traditionally-carved Jack-O-Lantern so it looked as if it was bursting through the pumpkin's temple. (The inspiration for this macabre piece of art came from a "Calvin and Hobbes" cartoon, a comic strip which I dearly miss.) On November 1st, I tried cooking the squash; it had a flavor and texture of a baked, damp cork.

On another occasion, a volunteer squash grew conveniently from the front corner of the compost bin. It yielded a pair of fruits that were too small and solid to be considered food (I had learned that lesson) but still sported attractive orange and green coloring which made for fine fall decorations.

This season the dilemma was a bit different. First of all, these volunteers were not growing out of the compost bin but were situated squarely in the middle of the new bed, a location that my mental "master plan" had tagged for melons. I would have pulled them for this reason alone, save for the fact that the two plants—which were starting to take on characteristics of a summer squash hybrid (no vine, unlike most winter squash that I know)—were five times the size of the zucchini squash that I had planted from store-bought seeds and were growing just a couple feet away. To even admit that I was struggling to grow zucchini—the low bar of gardening success (besides arugula)—was mortifying, but the truth sat there in the soil, along with pitiful bonsai versions of yellow crookneck and patty pan squashes. The vigorous volunteers, with their roots deep in nutrient-laden compost—showed signs that they would be producing fruit before the end of May. The good news was that I would actually have a chance to sample these Mendelian experiments in time to know whether I should pull them or transplant them before they cast too much shade over the young melon seedlings.

I have read about squash and squash-like plants of different species cross-pollinating to produce a toxic offspring, but really, are there truly any documented cases of poisoning by pumpkin? And if someone did admit themselves into a hospital with abdominal "discomfort," would they actually confess that it came as a result of eating a mystery vegetable from their garden?

The Hori Hori

Pacifists speak of turning swords into plowshares. This is all fine and good, but I think something exciting is lost when you convert a vorpal blade into a mundane garden trowel. Some tools even resent this reassignment and long for their former military careers. Robert Frost learned this the hard way and wrote about one such disgruntled, unemployed garden hoe:

> *But was there a rule*
> *The weapon should be*
> *Turned into a tool?*
> *And what do we see?*
> *The first tool I step on*
> *Turned into a weapon.*[2]

There certainly are tools that maintain their form, if not their function, from more aggressive times. Who has not launched a pitchfork into a leaf pile, emulating a Greek warrior wielding Poseidon's trident? Sadly, such displays of battle skills are rarely useful in the garden setting. But I am pleased to share with gardeners that there is at least one glorious exception: the hori hori. If this sounds to you like a ninja gardener's implement of destruction, then you're right. A horticultural utensil of Japanese origin, my own hori hori is a six-inch, slightly concave piece of stainless steel attached to a wooden hilt. It is a gardener's dagger, and it is nearly indestructible, entirely useful, and wicked-awesome. With it I can dig, weed, transplant, till, and in my spare time, whirl around and hurl it, end-over-end into the unassuming flesh of a discarded Jack O'Lantern. One edge of the blade is even serrated, so if my leg were to become pinned by a fallen corn stalk, and no one could hear my piteous calls for help, and if my cell phone battery was dead, I could, if necessary, use my hori hori

---

2. "My Objection to Being Stepped On" from a 1957 Christmas card (New York: Spiral Press).

to saw off my own limb to escape. Then I would use my hori hori to gently unearth a carrot to nurse myself back to health.

Never the Same Garden Twice

Organic gardeners talk about strategically utilizing plants and animals in a series of carefully orchestrated checks and balances that sounds so great when you read about it. Ladybugs eat aphids. Marigolds discourage white flies. Daffodils, when planted in a ring at the drip-line of your fruit trees, will discourage gophers. Put all of the pieces in place, and over the course of a calendar year you get a wonderful jigsaw puzzle image of a garden of flowers, bees, and a cornucopia of fruits and vegetables that is reassembled annually.

Not in my yard.

I was that kid who was always losing puzzle pieces.

I am beginning to think of my garden as more like the river that is never the same each moment and chooses a different channel every few years. There are constants, of course. The zucchini flowers will always attract squash bees; hornworms will always find the tomatoes. Groundsel will prevail as the dominant weed of the fall, followed by petty spurge in winter, and bindweed in summer. But other garden goings-on do not have such a regular pattern. One year, the gophers decimated my potatoes, but the following year they ignored them completely, despite being planted in the exact same place. Peppers produced a bumper crop in 2009, but the same variety forgot they were supposed to turn red in 2011. In 2013, shallow containers of beer became the final resting place for millipedes but no slugs. My seedlings still got eaten, however—I went out at 1 a.m. to determine that the culprit was an army of earwigs. One spring, hundreds of little green caterpillars that I had never seen in previous seasons made dinner salad of one of my pear trees. After three weeks, they suddenly disappeared (along with 40% of the tree's foliage). The other two pear trees—different varieties—were completely untouched despite growing less than three feet from their less fortunate neighbor. Sunflowers sprouted amidst the front yard landscaping for the three consecutive years and then became suddenly absent. Similarly, pungent feverfew was once a dominant, unsolicited force in my yard, reseeding itself at will. Bristly, blue-flowering borage has now taken over this role.

Certainly the machinations of my family are significant, but far from lasting. For example, we can choose where to place eggplant starts or where to plant a fruit tree. But when we attempt to enforce our desires on a large scale, it is like trying to hold back the ocean. I sprinkled marigold seeds in every garden bed in an attempt to protect my plants from white flies, but in the end, only two "islands" of marigold managed to germinate and become established. Our efforts to exterminate bedstraw, the sticky seeds of which are the bane of dogs and dog owners, had the reverse outcome. Over the course of two years, we worked to uproot, trample, or bury bedstraw at every opportunity, but we found that such a task was like trying to shut down Michael Jordan in his prime. You can't stop it; you can only hope to contain it.

Peas, Please

"Please plant peas," requested my wife.

Granting her wish, I planted a packet in February 2008—a cute, yellow-podded variety that I found in a seed catalog. They sprouted, the slugs and snails gorged, and I planted again. Five plants survived and started producing peas by mid-April. They yielded about three handfuls of tasty, if diminutive, yellow pea pods before the summer heat arrived and the plants shut down. I saved some seeds.

"Actually, dear, I prefer green peas."

Oh . . .

So the next year I planted green peas and started them in late January. The slugs and snails got fat again, and I replanted twice. By March, I saw flowers, and I was able to harvest young snow peas for about three weeks (six good handfuls) before the plants began to slow down.

"Actually, dear, my favorite are sugar snap peas."

So I started planting again the following January—just sugar snap peas—and also made a mental note that the previous year's snow peas had reseeded, sending out young sprouts the previous November. By February, these snow peas were twice as big as my slug-ravaged snap peas despite the "beer traps" that I had carefully set out. With the help of my then 1½-year-old daughter, we harvested four handfuls each of snap peas and snow peas.

I also noticed that my snap peas were significantly smaller, slimmer, and not as sweet as those at the farmers' market. It was not until the end of the season that I learned a key to bigger, tastier peas is to leave them on the vine longer.

My wife noticed, too.

"Would you plant more peas next year, dear? And did I mention that I'm not as big a fan of the snow peas?"

So that fall I bought two packages of sugar snap peas and set them in the soil in November after the second big autumn rain. My daughter, now two and a half, started picking them in the spring as soon as they were identifiable as pea pods. We had five good weeks of pea harvest.

"Could you plant more peas next year dear? And it would be great to have them closer to the house."

This past year on Thanksgiving, I sowed three packages of sugar snap peas in half of a new raised bed located just off the back patio. In the other half of the bed, I planted parsley and carrots. My daughter and I waited patiently for the pea pods to plump up. They did great. We picked peas for the entire month of April and a week into May. The parsley and carrots did not fare as well.

"Those peas were terrific! Would you plant more of them next year?"

I plan to buy stock in sugar snap pea seeds. In the late fall, I will sow the entire bed with them; the parsley and carrots can live somewhere else.

Thoughts on Vertical Gardening

Another gardening "buzz phrase" is the "vertical garden," the idea that you can trellis an entire buffet's worth of fresh veggies on a plot of dirt the size of a kiddie pool, but extending ten feet into the air. Melons, tomatoes, pumpkins, and string beans droop off this tower of healthfulness like a vegetarian's version of the candy room in *Willie Wonka and the Chocolate Factory.*

Or something like that.

My dream was a bit simpler. I envisioned an 8-foot-high wall of cucumbers, providing salad fodder while at the same time extending afternoon shade to an outdoor dining area.

After two attempts, I am now concluding that this does not work in Chico, at least not for cucumbers. It seems our afternoon sun is too hot, and the vines stalled out in mid-July after hitting about four feet in height. My "wall of foliage" droops in the heat and looks like someone's sad attempt to toilet paper my garden with green-brown tissues.

Don't get me wrong. I have had success with vertical gardening in Chico. For those that want to try it, I would suggest Armenian cucumber (a type of melon that is eaten like a cucumber), Trombetta di Albenga summer squash, gourds, cherry tomatoes (just keep tying them to your trellis), or pole beans.

But leave the cucumbers on the horizontal.

Staying Whole

I know that, economically and environmentally speaking, gardening at my house is not a sustainable enterprise. When you add up the cost of seeds and gardening equipment, my inefficient water use, the amount of time that is required to care for the plants (till, plant, water, harvest), and the fact that the fruits of my labors are essentially going towards feeding just four people, the whole project must be considered more as a hobby rather than as a fully successful exercise in self-sufficiency. I am also quite aware that when I go to the farmers' markets, I can purchase reasonably priced veggies that are usually just as tasty, almost as local, equally as organic, and are grown with more environmental and economic efficiency than what I can manage in my backyard. Perhaps this will change as I gain more gardening wisdom and experience, but I doubt it.

But while my garden may not be sustainable in an easily quantifiable manner, I firmly believe that it is in a qualitative sense. You see, I enjoy gardening. I enjoy the feeling of being linked to my backyard and the plants and animals that live there, of recognizing how the aroma of the soil varies when it is hot or cool, noting the traffic of insects that zip around the sunflowers, and having the ability to pluck a cherry tomato off the vine and pop it directly into my mouth. I always leave my garden with a greater sense of peace than when I entered it. Eating meals that include produce from the yard becomes a more connected, intimate experience, because not only do I know where my food came from, but I also know that I was a part of that process.

In his book *The Last Child in the Woods*, Richard Louv points out that Chinese Taoists created gardens and greenhouses over 2,000 years ago for their health benefits. As for the Western world, as early as 1699 the book, *The English Gardener*, advised that one spend "spare time in the garden, either digging, setting out, or weeding; there is no better way to preserve your health."

In short, having a garden and being outside are things that sustain me. They help make me whole. This is my greatest justification for being an advocate for gardening—we need more whole people in the world.

The No-Harvest Garden

Move over flowering pear and ornamental cherry. In case you haven't heard, non-fruiting trees are now passé.

Non-fruiting trees are popular for their ornamental charm and tidy upkeep. Now however, I am pleased to report that I have perfected the ideal complement to the fruitless orchard: the no-harvest garden.

Come over to my yard where you can see and experience an entire garden of vegetables plants that never produce vegetables! That's right. Plenty of beautiful flowers and foliage from all of your summer favorites—tomatoes, cucumbers, peppers, tomatillos—but with none of the fuss of actually having to harvest or prepare any of them. Why? Because they just aren't there!

One bed is a sea of cucumber leaves dappled with exquisite yellow flowers; but do not despair—no hidden cucumbers have taken shelter beneath the foliage. You say you want to keep up with the (Farmer) Joneses, but heirloom tomatoes aren't your thing? Here in the corner are four non-fruiting tomato bushes, verdant enough to make your neighbors believe that you have the greenest thumb in the world. You don't even have to worry about tomato hornworms with these babies, because with no fruit on the plant, who cares! While you are at it, don't forget to get some bonsai-sized, no-mess, no-fruit peppers and eggplants. They will take as much or as little water as you want to give them, but they won't get any bigger, and best of all, they won't produce fruit!

So come on down to my garden! These plants are for sale and going fast. Or, if you're depressed because you actually want tomatoes but your plants just aren't putting out no matter how much you fertilize, water, and plead with them, then just take a stroll among my beds, and you will quickly feel much better in knowing that you are not alone. Admission is just $2.00.

Plant 'em Deep

A colleague of mine told me that last summer, he didn't water his tomatoes.

"Not a drop."

Huh?

"I planted each one in a pit" he said.

Huh?

"And I created drought-tolerant tomatoes."

Huh?

He described his method to me (it sounded much more promising than my attempts at vertical gardening), and here is what he did: In early April, he dug holes in the damp spring soil, each over a foot deep, and planted a tomato in each, leaving a good eight to twelve inches between the top of the leaves and the top of the hole. Then he placed a piece of glass over each hole to protect the plants from frost. As the tomato plants stretched to reach for the top of the hole, he would slowly add soil, thus encouraging roots to grow along the lengthening stems. By late May, the holes were all filled in, the glass removed, the tomato leaves were above grade, and each plant had a root system extending over a foot down into the earth. With the roots that deep, the plants were able to access enough water to sustain themselves through the summer and produce tomatoes straight through to October.

Little Neglected Plant Makes Good: A True Story of Floral Inspiration

In the farthest corner of the yard exists a spineless yucca, an otherworldly jungle of a plant that resembles a cross between an octopus and a Truffula tree. Overgrown limbs reach out from underneath the neighbor's pear tree and creep over a sagging pergola that is in desperate need of repair. Beneath the branches, all is shadows and cobwebs. Dust-covered brown leaves litter the crushed-granite soil, the last remnant of the previous owner's attempt to establish a xeriscape (cactus and the like), which seems strange to me in a region that gets an average of 26 inches of rain a year.

Yet despite the apparent inhospitability of this neglected part of the yard, a friend once commented about the "energy" he felt there. I raised my internal eyebrow at the time, but I have since retreated from my skepticism, mostly because of a single plant that called these shadows home for its first few years of life. Picture the floral version of *Slum Dog Millionaire*.

All I know is that some sort of energy allowed this one particular seed to sprout and grow. When I first noticed it, the isolated plant had about five leaves on long stems, rising vase-like about eight inches high. The leaves were a dusky dark green, fuzzy, and palmate. One year later, the plant looked exactly the same, as if frozen in time, unaffected by rain, frost, sun, or insects.

However, by now some pioneering weeds—grasses and lamb's quarters—were beginning to establish outposts among the gravel, and a cardboard plus woodchip weed-smothering project was on the horizon. Not wishing to bury "Little Fuzzy" along with the weeds, I transplanted it to a sunny spot near the entrance of my garden, gave it a dowsing of water as an apology for displacing it, and watched as four of its five leaves promptly drooped and shriveled away.

One leaf remained. I thought the end was near, and it was destined to follow in the footsteps of so many other well-intentioned failures. Yet, a week later I noticed a small, new leaf emerging from the center of the plant. Then came a third and fourth, and by mid-spring a bouquet of basal leaves covered a 2.5-foot-diameter area and warranted rerouting of the garden path. May arrived, and a stalk began extending from the middle of the greenery, and only then was I able to impress my neighbors by ceasing to use the moniker of "unknown fuzzy-leafed thing" and upgrade to the more common name: hollyhock. The stalk eventually sky-scrapered to eight feet with hot pink flowers that lasted well into October.

Eventually the plant died, but it left its legacy for years to come. The flowers gave way to dry donut-shaped fruits, the seeds inside were arranged like slides in an old-fashioned carousel. Wind, birds, and footsteps scattered the black seeds around the yard. The following year another hollyhock spire grew adjacent to the peach tree. It produced multiple stalks for two seasons before I finally pulled out a dried root ball six inches thick. This past summer four hollyhocks could be seen flowering in various parts of the yard, where they served as popular stops for carpenter bees, which flew away with a comical dusting of yellow pollen clinging to their jet-black bodies.

It is November 1st as I type this, and still the flowers linger.

CHAPTER 3

Overland Migratory Gophers (OMGs) & Other Critters

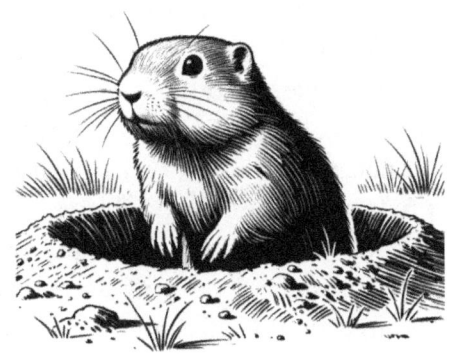

Snails, Slugs, and Gophers

Snails are the only creatures in the garden that truly fear me. Ever since I busted out the escargot recipe, they haven't presented too much of a problem. At the end of two weeks of "collecting," I had placed nearly 100 slimers in a plastic bin lined with cornmeal. While this gastronomic experiment eventually ended up as a soil amendment, the resulting impact on the snail population was substantial.

But then there are the slugs. Like the coyotes that became top dog in Yellowstone after the wolf population was wiped out, the slugs now pretty much have free rein over all my young sprouts. Additionally, I have four raised beds constructed out of reclaimed "urbanite"—concrete chunks of ripped-up patio—which contain cracks that provide ample housing opportunities for the one-inch mollusks. Creating slug habitat was not my intent when I made those beds. Chalk this one up to an eco-idea from some well-intentioned internet article that I should have more thoroughly vetted prior to implementation. Fortunately, these crevices are also ideal for a new friend of mine, the alligator lizard. Between the lizards and shallow containers of cheap beer, I have been able to keep the slugs at bay, but there is still a lot of seedling carnage that takes place in April.

I do wish the alligator lizards were a bit bigger and had a taste for gopher flesh. Poisons and traps are not really my style, and the "flooding" method didn't work (I thought I saw one gopher with swim trunks and a snorkel). Also, unlike the other garden pests, local gophers are native; they were here long before Europeans arrived with their zucchini and carrot crops. So naturally, the best way to control them would be to introduce a native predator. It would be hard to train a hawk to limit its meals to the morsels that can only be found on my property, so perhaps a snake or two? I have considered carrying an empty burlap sack when I go hiking in the foothills on the off-chance I come across a gopher snake that is interested in relocating, all expenses paid, to my backyard.

Then there is gopher spurge. Spurge is a plant (*Euphorbia* sp.) that has a milky sap which stains and chaps the skin and, if you are unlucky enough to have some splash into your face (like me), burns your eyeballs in fiery agony for a couple hours. No fewer than four species of euphorbia grow annually in my yard. The wisdom is that gophers won't eat it, so in theory, you can plant a border of spurge around your plants as a deterrent. One year I planted said botanical moat, and I found out it is true—gophers won't eat the spurge. But they still got to my tomatoes. It didn't take the gophers long to figure out that it was possible to go under or around the spurge rather than through it.

For the first few years of living in Chico I didn't have much of a problem with gophers; I think in part because the previous owners had a couple of cats and three dogs, so I guess the rodents knew better. But they weren't very intimidated by our family's half-blind, 12-year-old terrier. I have found that the only thing that really seems to have a real effect is lining all gardening areas with wire mesh (a.k.a. "hardware cloth"), and even that isn't always 100% perfect. But as with everything, the gophers have their place. This past winter I constructed a bomb-proof garden box, a 13-inch high, 14-foot long wooden structure, the bottom and sides lined with ½" wire mesh. While the plants inside are safe, this has not diminished the spirit of the gophers, one of which has taken up residence beneath the mesh. One morning the gopher treated my daughter and I to a mini wild animal show, and for 15 minutes we stared at the ground in anticipation, both of us entranced as we watched the critter tentatively poking out of its hole as it diligently cleared soil from its tunnel beneath the bed. That evening I added two shovelfuls of the freshly tilled dirt to box above.

Eulogy for a Bantam

A number of years ago I woke up to the sound of a rooster in the backyard. This was odd because we didn't own a rooster. When I heard it again a few seconds later, I went out to investigate, expecting to find some wayward cock-a-doodle on our side of the fence, perhaps trying to create a live-action version of the movie *Chicken Run*. But instead of a long-tailed fowl, I spied our four-year-old bantam hen perched authoritatively on top of the coop. It couldn't be her, I thought. She eyed me as I approached, and after a few moments she let out a wail. Not quite your classic rooster crow—a bit shorter and perhaps a slightly higher pitch—but pretty darn close. She continued to serenade the neighborhood each morning for the next few weeks, eventually tapering off her efforts. After a three-year hiatus, she did it again.

Her name was Bitsy. She was part of our first foray into chicken ownership, along with ten additional fluffy chicks that would grow into standard-sized hens. Bitsy was an "Old English Bantam," essentially, a small brown bird about one-third the size of a normal chicken. It has been said that a farm is not complete without a pig. I would suggest that a backyard chicken flock is not complete without a banty.

I have read that the bantam breeds are a product of the Industrial Revolution. As people moved from the country into the cities to work in the factories, they still wanted access to fresh eggs, so they took their birds with them. The chickens were bred to be small to accommodate city life and apartment living as bantams need much less space and food than larger birds. Picture chicken enclosures in alleyways or on apartment balconies.

I pause here to apologize to those readers who think that this—an essay about a pet chicken—is beyond cliché. You may be sick of wannabe farmer-authors waxing poetic about their flock and the novel idiosyncrasies of each and every hen or rooster that (so they would have you believe) also serve indispensable ecological, spiritual, and culinary roles in the family homestead, all the while contributing to the collective Chi of Mother

Earth. But this story is not some drawn-out meme intended to amuse and elicit a "Like," and it does not have a happy ending. Memes are there for a few days or weeks at most, and then they are gone. Bitsy was the opposite. The word I would use to describe her was "present."

She was present at my daughters' preschool show-and-tells, as well as for multiple semesters in my introductory life science classes where she served as a focal point for lessons on evolution, natural selection, and selective breeding.

She was present not only in the chicken coop, but in our entire yard. Being lighter and more nimble than the other birds, she had no problem flapping over the six-foot high wire fence that enclosed the run. She roamed the property freely, scratching the ground for insects or nipping off pieces of kale, undeterred by squirrels, scrub jays, or our two dogs. For a few weeks at a time, she would refuse to roost in the coop, preferring instead to set up camp in the branches of the elderberry shrub nearby.

Most notably, she was present in our family stories. I won't go into the details—every pet has their special quirky moments that are usually a hundred times more meaningful to the owners than they are to the public (think YouTube cat videos). Suffice it to say, Bitsy's adventures, both real and fictitious, were shared repeatedly around the dinner table and at bedtime. The stories became lore, and then legend, as special to our daughters as any fairytale or Shel Silverstein poem.

Our original flock was purchased at the end of the summer of 2013. One of the first lessons you learn when you own chickens is that they are not the hardiest of pets. They succumb to raccoons, infection, heat stroke, terriers, and (rarely) old age. We try to give each bird the best life that they can have, but my family quickly grew to understand that death happens.

I have dug over a dozen holes in the backyard over the past decade, creating a veritable poultry cemetery of unmarked graves. We replenish the flock with baby chicks every three to four years, about six birds at a time, different breeds, different colors. When I look into the coop now, it is hard to remember which bird is from what cohort. We always believed that Bitsy's adventuresome spirit would likely lead to an abbreviated existence.

We were quite wrong. She outlived every member of the original flock. And most of the second cohort. And even some of the third.

She started crowing again for the third time at the beginning of October 2022. And then, on the morning of the 19th, there was silence. Bitsy was nowhere to be found.

A text message was sent to the neighbors asking them to keep their eyes open. We got a response that evening, and subsequently we were sadly presented with Bitsy's leg reverently wrapped in a paper towel. The neighbor said her dog had brought it from the yard, but it was clear that the pooch had simply been a courier and not the responsible party. As for the rest of Bitsy, we never found a trace, not even a feather. I guessed that a cat, or perhaps a hawk, had been part of the final chapter of her life.

I'll save the sappy "Circle of Life" parable for the other chickens that have died over the years, interred at the base of fruit trees or deep beneath garden beds. Those eulogies have become brief and predictable as my family gives appreciation for each hen's companionship and contribution during its life, and we take what comfort we can in knowing their bodies will be recycled into oak branches, lavender blossoms, and summer vegetables. But this is not how we think of Bitsy. She was more than a niche in the ecology of the garden. She was part of the growth of our family. The last surviving member of our original flock of birds, she lived for over nine years. For perspective, at the time this accounted for two-thirds of the life of our older daughter and more than three quarters of the life of our younger daughter.

Bitsy will be missed. With her gone, our yard is noticeably emptier, and quieter, and we are sad.

Wigging Out

I scribbled down this nugget of wisdom on a piece of paper entitled "Notes for 2020 Garden": *"Everything from starts. No exceptions—<u>Earwigs</u>."* Yes, earwigs. I used to think they were just an unpleasant reality of growing chard, where they hide in the deep, protective crevices between the stem and the base of each leaf. But a wet winter and spring proved me wrong. I saw them everywhere, and they went "full buffet" on my garden, gorging on pea shoots, bean leaves, artichokes, and sunflowers, especially the young, tender plants. I set out traps of cheap beer and vegetable oil. The brew lured only a handful, and the vegetable oil was ineffective. More satisfying was a nightly ritual of hunting them with a flashlight and then spraying them with a toxic 50-50 blend of water and rubbing alcohol, but after a couple of weeks I realized I wasn't even making a dent in the population, and the chore quickly became tiresome. Eventually I accepted the losses, replanted, and moved on.

Earwigs are native to Europe, and were first observed in California in 1923. They are omnivores, except in my yard, where they seem to be strict vegetarians. I read that they especially like moisture and mild weather—in other words, Chico, Spring 2019. After I had seeded my bean row for a third time, I went onto the internet and determined a plan if the earwigs become a problem in a future year. Yes, dear readers, earwigs are edible and nutritious. Stay tuned.

Observations II

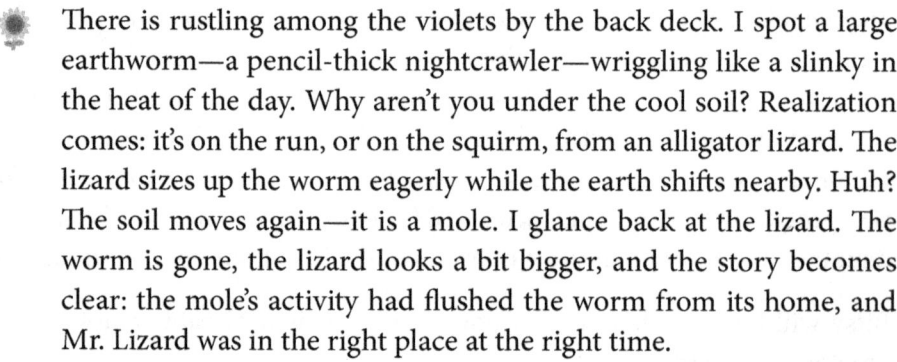
- There is rustling among the violets by the back deck. I spot a large earthworm—a pencil-thick nightcrawler—wriggling like a slinky in the heat of the day. Why aren't you under the cool soil? Realization comes: it's on the run, or on the squirm, from an alligator lizard. The lizard sizes up the worm eagerly while the earth shifts nearby. Huh? The soil moves again—it is a mole. I glance back at the lizard. The worm is gone, the lizard looks a bit bigger, and the story becomes clear: the mole's activity had flushed the worm from its home, and Mr. Lizard was in the right place at the right time.

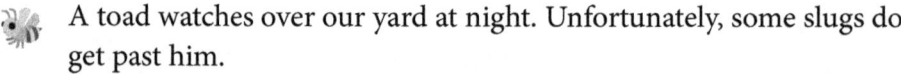
- A toad watches over our yard at night. Unfortunately, some slugs do get past him.

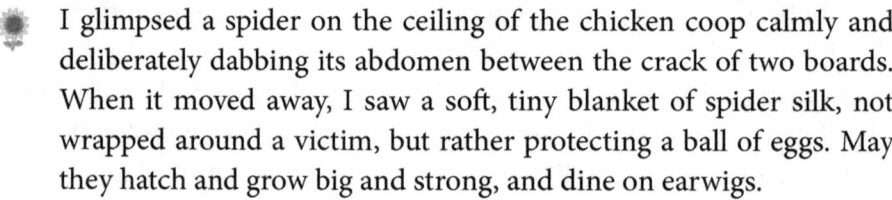
- I glimpsed a spider on the ceiling of the chicken coop calmly and deliberately dabbing its abdomen between the crack of two boards. When it moved away, I saw a soft, tiny blanket of spider silk, not wrapped around a victim, but rather protecting a ball of eggs. May they hatch and grow big and strong, and dine on earwigs.

As I was rescuing a young garlic stalk from the growing encroachment of some wood sorrel (clover-shaped leaves and little yellow flowers), I heard the familiar buzz of a honeybee nearby. It was not interested in the sorrel. Rather, its attention was, strangely, on the garlic. I watched the bee patiently. It landed at the base of a garlic leaf, where a half teaspoon's worth of sprinkler water had collected in the crevice between the leaf and the stem earlier that morning. Then the bee relaxed its wings, stuck out its tongue, and took a drink. Soon after I snapped my photo, it flew off to resume its more usual business.

 I heard a bird call from a tree in the neighbor's yard. It reminded me of being in a mountain campground among the pines. Birding field guides try to put into "words" what the bird vocalizations sound like, but I seriously believe something gets lost in translation. For example, I cannot recall a hummingbird chirping *"ZEE-chuppity-chup!"* Fortunately, the sound I heard was distinct and memorable enough that I was able to repeat it to a birding friend a couple days later. He suggested it was a White-Breasted Nuthatch. A few smartphone taps later, and I was listening to the nuthatch call, but it didn't sound quite right. "Perhaps a Red-Breasted Nuthatch?" he suggested. I consulted the internet again—Bingo! I learned that the Red-Breasted Nuthatch is a cute little bird that hops along tree trunks and will often retreat from the snowy mountains in the winter to spend time in the valley. Its call, according to the guide book, is *"yank yank yank."* Whatever.

How to Train Your Spider

"Now you're a curious looking critter." Such was my first innocent thought when I spotted a gray, ornately decorated insect perched on an unripe cherry tomato. Partially hidden by the dense foliage, it was handsome, as far as such creatures go, with a dusky white horizontal stripe across its back and leaf-like fins protruding from the lower part of its rear legs, which brought up images of the alien "bugs" from the B-movie *Starship Troopers*. It turns out it actually was a bug, a "true bug" in the scientific sense of the word. Unlike beetles, which have a larva which grow, form a chrysalis, and then eventually hatch into adults (like ladybugs), true bugs hatch from eggs and then remain six-legged creatures for the rest of their lives, growing to adulthood in series of stages, shedding their skin each time they get a little bigger. The specimen in my yard was a leaf-footed bug (*Leptoglossus* sp.), and it was not long before I had a chance to meet its entire family. Within a couple weeks I noted the red nymphs, or instars (a.k.a. baby leaf-footed bugs) and its brothers and sisters (and aunts and uncles and cousins), tiptoeing delicately over the cherry tomatoes. But they weren't just tiptoeing.

I had planted a substantial row of tomatoes of mixed varieties, so I was not too concerned when some of the cherry tomatoes began to look like they had the measles. There were plenty of tomatoes to go around, and I knew that even my family wouldn't be able to eat them faster than they ripened. Besides, I am a believer in the power of natural biological control, and I was sure something in my yard would find the leaf-footed bugs to be a tasty treat if they got too out of hand—perhaps birds, or a parasitic wasp, or some other cool critter mentioned in one of my partially-read gardening books. I kept a lookout for one creature in particular that I was hoping would help me out.

The first tomatoes to ripen are the cherries, and the larger varieties follow a few weeks later—Black Krims and Mortgage Lifters and others with similarly catchy names that had sounded worthy of purchase a few months prior. It was not long before these plants were also crawling with leaf-footed bugs. A small army of them had moved in, and they were literally sucking the juice out of my tomatoes, without the fear of predators that I hoped the "wildness" of my garden would bring. Instead, the leaf-footed bugs were as casual as cows grazing a pasture, and if I stuck my hand into the tomato thicket to harvest, they would simply side-step over to an adjacent fruit and the carnage would continue. Perhaps a third of each tomato was edible, if that. Where was my biological control? Where were the praying mantises, the black phoebes, and the parasitic wasps?

My savior—or so I hoped—appeared the first week of August. A more lyrical writer might have named her "Neoscona," but at the time I simply told my wife that the spider was back. I slept well that night, dreaming pleasantly of leaf-footed bugs unwittingly meandering into her web, forever leaving my tomatoes in peace.

Neoscona oaxacensis was likely one of the multitude of North American spiders collected in the late 1800s by the German–born arachnologist George Marx. Also called the Western Spotted Orb Weaver, it can be found from Peru all the way to eastern Washington state. Though I am sure it is a year-round resident in my yard, it seems to emerge from nowhere in the latter half of the summer, making a glorious entrance with a grand, spiraling web that often stretches four feet across, with anchor points even further out. It is, in my opinion, the iconic arachnid. It diligently spins or repairs its web, as needed, once a day, a beautiful geometric tapestry that this particular summer stretched lavishly between a tomato cage and a nearby crepe myrtle, a total span of nearly 10 feet. With its legs extended, the spider measured two inches from front leg to back leg, with a robust decorated brown and yellow abdomen and pronounced fangs. It would be the perfect weapon against the leaf-footed bugs.

Each day I carefully ducked under the web as I waited for the spider to make an impact. And I waited. Its net trapped many insects—small flies, a ladybug, and even a honeybee, but I never saw a single leaf-footed bug. By summer's end, all of my tomato plants had been reduced to fruitless shrubbery.

Lessons learned: 1) Dense foliage on tomato plants is the perfect habitat for leaf-footed bugs (and other critters). Liberally pruning the leaves is recommended. 2) That same summer my daughter had her own tomato plants in the ground twelve feet away, separated from my plants by two hearty zucchini vines. Her tomatoes were minimally impacted by the bugs, which pretty much liked to stay on a single plant. The takeaway is that it is a good idea to scatter your tomatoes throughout the yard, which can limit the damage. 3) Spiders are hard to train.

Praying Mantis

The praying mantis is one of the most fascinating creatures in our yard. Early in the summer we may catch a fleeting glimpse of newly hatched mantises, each one not much bigger than an ant, scampering with the speed of spiders to hide among the lemon balm leaves. Their vulnerability is evident, and for six weeks they abruptly seem to disappear entirely—I am sure the vast majority become part of the food chain. But come late July, I will casually gaze up the stalk of a sunflower and find a four-inch long green or brown adult mantis clinging patiently to the edge of the flower waiting for a meal. The quick nervousness of its youth is gone; it is now a top predator of the garden. It does not run from potential danger and prefers now to blend into the background, or perhaps allow its spines and alien visage to make even the scrub jays think twice about turning it into a snack.

Over the course of a week, I will find two or three more but that's it. Each has its own sunflower plant and can often be found in the same place on the same flower head for many days in a row. For the longest time I wondered why I had never actually seen one eat, for certainly it must take a lot of meals to create a creature so large in such a short time. Then one day I happened to come across a mantis halfway through lunch—a bee—and ten seconds later it was over. The dining speed of this creature would give Coney Island hot-dog eating contestants a run for their money and is just as captivating—if not nauseating—to watch. The difference was the mantis did not end up with a distended belly. It merely wiped at its face a few times with its long forelegs before taking five calm, measured steps to the other side of the flower, where it again began the patient wait for its next meal to arrive.

Vacancy

"Your yard is already home to insects galore, so why not give bees a proper place to rest their wings? Bee hotels, also called nests or houses, are a great way to attract pollinators to your family's flower or vegetable garden." ~National Geographic website

Yes, this is the essay on bee hotels. You might have guessed this was coming. It doesn't take long before a gardener stumbles upon an article for a bee hotel, possibly on the internet, or on the cover of a sustainable living magazine. One sees these insect chalets every now and again, often at the native plant garden outside of a science museum or nature center. There is a large one adjacent to the Organic Vegetable Project at the CSU Chico University Farm.

Magazine articles about them remind the reader that the Eurasian honeybees can only do so much pollinating, and we can't forget the role that native bees play. Honeybees didn't even arrive in California until the 1700s, when they were introduced by the Spanish to support the agricultural efforts of the missions. Until then, the native bees did all the work. Native California bees, of which there are over 1,600 species, include mason bees, sweat bees, bumblebees, carpenter bees, and more. They do not make hives like honeybees. Rather, they are solitary, and find cracks, crevices, and holes in wood, rocks, bark, sand, or mud in which they lay their eggs and rear their young. And—according to apiaphiles everywhere—you can give them a hand by building your very own bee hotel.

I admit it. I got suckered.

But who wouldn't? Do a search for "bee hotel images" and you will see what I mean. They look soooo elegant, so natural, so simple. Bee hotels are functional pieces of art made from material found in nature. They have the same appeal as wicker chairs, Christmas wreaths, or bird houses. They are diverse in size and shape and texture. Lastly, they don't seem very complicated to make (Read: Famous last words).

I speculated that the ideal place for a bee hotel would be adjacent to a native plant garden in an urban setting where more space is taken up by concrete sidewalks than soil and foliage, and proper habitat for native bees is in short supply. The irony here is that this does not describe my property at all. There are cracks and crevices everywhere in my yard—in rotting stumps, discarded playground sand, soil, compost, tree bark, rock walls, and spaces between the house siding, just to name a few. And native bees are plentiful as well.

So why did I want a bee hotel? Certainly for my benefit, not for the bees. In addition to the aesthetic attributes, my family had never actually seen a baby bee emerge from a crevice, flex its new wings, and fly off on its maiden voyage. Butterflies and birds yes, but not bees.

So I built one—roughly 2 feet by 2 feet, 7.5 inches deep, with a nice sloped triangular roof, complete with real roofing material. The hotel was partitioned into ten "rooms," six below and four smaller ones in the "attic." I collected pine cones and chunks of tree bark. I drilled holes in logs and hollowed out dozens of elderberry stems. I carefully filled each "room" with a different material, and when I was done my hotel had hundreds of crevices from which the bees could choose, everything ranging from the single occupancy economy holes to the deluxe suite (multiple holes drilled into the shape of a heart). A last, late addition to the hotel was a wire screen. This was recommended by several websites to keep birds from mistaking the bee hotel for a snack dispenser. The downside was that it made the edifice look more like an insect penitentiary than a 5-star Marriott. This was not the bee hotel that would make the cover of a magazine.

At the end of March, I situated my creation against the fence on the west side of the yard, open to the east to catch the morning sun but avoid the afternoon heat. It was too heavy to actually mount onto the fence, so I placed it up on cinder blocks to get it off the dirt, though this was not enough to raise it to the recommended height of 3 to 5 feet, which apparently best accommodates the flight path of the bees (this is a project for a later date). At least the attic rooms were roughly three feet above the ground.

And then I waited.

A few spiders moved in first, including a black widow. I saw a slug one evening. The summer dust and pollen accumulated on the spider webs and pine cones, and soon the entire structure started looking less like a whimsical work of art and more like a dreary miniature version of the Addams Family Mansion.

It wasn't until well into the fall that I spied little plugs of dried mud in three of the drilled holes, evidence of mason bees. There might have been more, but I fear that a number of potential tenants had been eaten by the spiders soon after their arrival. The following April I noticed two plugs were askew, the third was gone. A bit anticlimactic—I had imagined that the bees' emergence would have been heralded by inspirational music magically emanating from the hotel, but hey, I'll call it a success.

The spiders, meanwhile, haven't paid their rent in weeks.

Pollination Appreciation

I have taken some time to really notice the myriad of pollinating insects going about their business around my yard. I highly recommend it. I am amazed not only by their numbers—the buzzing of the activity around the catmint blooms (*Nepeta* sp.) can be especially loud—but also by their diversity.

In addition to the catmint, a rainbow of other flowers including daisies, lilies, bindweed, sunflowers, yarrow, poppies, rosemary, and squash blossoms boosts the variety of pollinators on our property. On a typical June afternoon, we will see honeybees, bumblebees, wasps, hoverflies, bee flies, hummingbirds, butterflies, and more. Not only do certain species prefer certain plants, but also different times of day. The giant black carpenter bee[1] ventures out to the larkspur in the late afternoon, while moths come by the lavender once the sun has set to pick over whatever pollen scraps were left behind by the honeybees.

I bring my face inches from a bumblebee and admire its efforts with wonder and appreciation.

Owl Box

Over the years I've built a chicken coop (success!), a bee hotel (success!—if you don't mind spiders instead of bees), and a compost pile (home for decomposing yard trimmings, pill bugs, centipedes, and rats, so, another success!). My track record of building habitats is unblemished! Not to rest on my laurels, I pondered my next project—an owl box. It would be my Frank Lloyd Wright moment: I pictured a mated pair of Great Horned Owls 40 feet up a tree, rearing their young, and keeping watch over the property while perched on the front porch of an owl chalet that I had constructed.

In addition to exercising my carpentry muscles and adding more charismatic megafauna to my property, I had a third reason to build an owl box: I was fed up with gophers and moles creating a subway system below the garden and lawn. I had contemplated "relocating" a wild gopher snake

---

1. The less commonly seen male Valley Carpenter Bee is orange with striking green eyes. One is pictured on the back cover.

to my yard on more than one occasion, but it's probably illegal, and there would be no guarantee it would do what I asked (refer to "How to Train Your Spider"). Over the years, we have heard the calls of Western Screech-Owls, Great Horned Owls, and American Barn Owls in our neighborhood. My family had also recently seen the film *The Biggest Little Farm* in which the owners put up dozens of owl boxes on their 200-acre farm, attracting 87 barn owls that consumed tens of thousands of gophers a year. And I only needed to attract one family of owls.

I took inventory of my random lumber supply and limited tools. I had plywood, a circular saw (a 40+ year-old hand-me-down from my father), a drill, hammer, nails, screws, and plenty of Gorilla Glue. Yep, I thought. I can make this work.

But the devil is in the details. First, location. Did I even have a place for an owl box? The most promising site was up high on the side of a redwood tree, but that spot was currently home to an occupied bat box. Could one be mounted above the other? After reflection, I recalled that owls have been known to eat bats, so probably not a great idea. A young 18-inch diameter oak on the other side of the property was the next best option. While it did not have the benefit of providing the same cover and natural year-round shade as an evergreen tree, it would probably suffice. I had, after all, seen photos of owl boxes mounted on poles at the edge of orchards where there is no cover at all.

Then I looked at plans for owl boxes. Apparently, there are a lot of right ways to do it, and a lot of wrong ways. For example, owl boxes that are designed to be mounted under the eave of a barn are, by definition, protected from weather and are thus constructed much differently from those meant to be attached to a tree where they are exposed to the elements. There is no barn on my property. I looked again at my lumber options and realized that the sheet of plywood that I had planned to use was actually low-grade strand board, and it dawned on me that it probably wouldn't survive a single rainstorm, much less multiple winters. Additional research revealed that the glue used in strand board usually contains formaldehyde, so not only would the owls get wet, they would be poisoned too.

So a purchase of high-grade cedar or redwood boards was going to be needed. This meant I really needed to know what I was doing, which is a problem for a "measure once, cut twice, and use some glue and duct tape" kind of guy. But the final nail in the coffin of my mind's-eye masterpiece (before I even had a chance to swing my hammer) was the photo on the internet of a dead baby owl at the base of a tree, the result—according to the website—of a poorly constructed owl box.

I think I will ask for a prefabricated owl box for my birthday.

OMG

"Overland migratory gophers," said Mark.

"Come again?"

"Pocket gophers, but they migrate overland, so I was told. They can go up and over the hardware cloth, so you need to make sure it rises high enough over the soil. At least four inches."

Most people would be dismayed by this news, especially someone like me whose hardware cloth peeks barely an inch above the garden bed in some places, but in fact I was overjoyed! I had yet another gardening excuse under my belt, one that was not only brilliant, but also rolled off the tongue in a manner worthy of the fine print in the Sunset Garden Guide. Go ahead and try it: "*My real challenge is the overland migratory pocket gophers, which are actually endemic to west Chico, California.*"

I don't even care if it is true; I intend to use it over and over.

The Center of the Garden

What is at the center of my garden? Not just the physical center, but the ecological center, the musical center, or the spiritual center? If the rainbow that I see in the misty spray of the garden hose were to form a complete circle, what would be in the middle? Contemporary research and thought about agriculture points to the soil, with its complex interactions and interplay between the organic and inorganic worlds: plant roots, fungal hyphae, bacteria, rocks, and minerals all intertwined on the macroscopic, microscopic, and atomic levels. Others suggest it is the seed, a complete package of nutrients and genetic material that allows a plant to germinate and grow into any myriad of forms depending on the instructions provided by the DNA—a stalk of corn, an apple tree, a Venus flytrap, or a rose. In the case of the Coast Redwood, a seed weighing approximately 1/3000 of an ounce can become the tallest organism on the planet, so big that its canopy provides an ecosystem unto itself. In the misty fog 250 feet above the forest floor, the crevices in and among the branches and trunk accumulate decades of redwood duff. Kept moist year-round by summer fog and winter rain, this organic matter provides a substrate for moss, ferns, huckleberry, and other plants. In this aerial habitat, one can find falcons, banana slugs, voles, and salamanders, which live their entire lives without ever touching the ground below. In my career as an outdoor educator, I have shared that water is the source of life, and that there is a type of magic that exists in the boomerang-shaped molecule of a single oxygen atom covalently bonded to two hydrogen atoms, one on each side. The water molecule's 104-degree angle is the key to its unique properties; this bend helps provide the molecule's polarity and, in turn, its reactivity— the chemical reactions of all life on the planet are guided by the atomic structure of water.

Soil, seed, water—a fine argument could be made for any one of these to be a reasonable answer to the question "What is at the center of my garden?" One might add air or sunlight to this list of viable responses. Yet, as I stroll out to get the mail on a cool day in early February, a break in the clouds releases the sunlight to shine on the row of rosemary limbs that creep through the fence and encroach on the sidewalk. The rosemary seems to be perpetually in bloom with light blue flowers, and, despite the chill, there is activity among the blossoms. I am talking, of course, of bees.

I believe that bees exist at the center of it all. Follow a honeybee around the yard, and you see how it is all connected—flower to flower, plant to plant, anther to stigma, the human world to the natural world. The bees provide a bridge between science that we understand and concepts which remain an amazing mystery.

For countless trees, shrubs, and herbs, the bee is integral to the lifecycle of the plant. A bee visiting one flower to gather nectar will invariably be dusted with pollen in the process. The pollen, which is the plant world's equivalent of sperm (technically "gametophyte"), will travel on the hairs of the bee to a nearby flower where the pollen brushes up against the flower's stigma, eventually leading to the fertilization of the plant's seeds. While bees are not the only creatures that pollinate flowers, they are known to be one of the most efficient. So important is this to the lives of plants that they have, over countless millennia, adapted numerous features to be more inviting to the bees. Showy, colorful flowers; fragrant, high-sugar nectar; and "landing pad" shaped blossoms are all examples of adaptations with the express purpose of attracting bees. There is even a European orchid species that mimics both the shape, and scent, of a female long-horned bee for the purpose of attracting male bees to the flower. One assumes that the male bee leaves disappointed in what it finds, departing only with some pollen dust as a consolation prize.

In my yard, the orange or yellow petals of the calendula bend gently into the shape of a parabola. Not only do the petals appear bright even in the winter, the flower's shape focuses the sunlight, nudging the temperature up by a degree or two, providing an extra element of warmth for the visiting bees. For tomato flowers, ideal pollination occurs when the vibration of the bee's wings comes into contact with the flower, which loosens the pollen. Some gardening guides suggest that in the absence of honeybees an electric toothbrush can be used. I tried this once and found it to be painstakingly tedious (and mostly ineffective), and my appreciation for the abilities of the bees increased even further.

And of course, while a bee might not be at the exact center of the web of life, they are part of the food web. Sometimes this web is quite literal as an unlucky bee finds itself stuck in one to become a meal for a garden spider, which in turn might find its way into the belly of a Scrub Jay.

From the human perspective, the importance of bees cannot be understated. Pollination leads to seeds, fruits, and nuts. An oft-quoted statistic states that, globally, one in every three bites of food eaten by humans owes its existence to bees. The breakfast cereal box has conditioned us to think of bees as the provider of honey, or perhaps the beeswax of the honeycomb, yet when compared to the importance of the global food supply, honey and wax become almost trivial.

But what kind of bees? Prior to the year 1600, the sunflowers and "Three Sisters" crops of corn, beans, and squash that were planted by the indigenous peoples of North America were not visited by the honeybees with which we are most familiar. Pollination instead was the role of hundreds of species of native, and mostly solitary bees, including carpenter bees, mason bees, bumblebees, and countless others.

Like most of you reading this, honeybees have immigrants in their ancestry. The honeybees that I see in my yard are native to the Old World. Cultivated since antiquity, European colonists introduced honeybees to the Americas during the 17th century. I mistakenly used to think of honeybees as a timeless element of California's ecology, as permanent as hawks and redwood trees, and yet the reality is that they represent a dynamic ecosystem that changes over time. Honeybees are part of a club of organisms—from dogs and rats to apples, Bermuda grass, cockroaches, and starlings—whose global existence is owed, in one way or another, to human exploration, ingenuity, ignorance, or carelessness. The extinction of the Passenger Pigeon, the mammoth, and countless other species show the other side of the changing ecosystem dominated by the impact of *Homo sapiens*.

Yet despite their Eurasian roots, honeybees do not have any prejudice toward the native plants in my yard—the flaming magenta blossoms of the native redbud get just as much attention as the delicate, diminutive, red and white flowers of the Japanese maple. Can one state that "All Plants Matter" to honeybees? Why not?

Honeybees have been long anthropomorphized to represent a broad range of emotions, activities, and virtues that are central to humanity. (The extreme example of bees being "gifted" with human attributes—including noses, smiles, and even a command of the English language—can be found in comedian Jerry Seinfeld's *Bee Movie*). Bees are industrious, dedicated workers, whether in search of nectar, building the honeycomb, or caring for their young. We admire them for their unwavering sense of purpose. They protect the hive and the queen with their lives if necessary. They can be graceful in flight, yet on more than one occasion I have observed a thumb-sized carpenter bee misjudge the weight-bearing ability of a flower only to find itself, and the flower petals, toppling to the ground before shakily flying off (though unlike humans, I don't believe the embarrassment lingered). And, similar to many people, the ire of bees can be unpredictable—I doubt that I am alone in feeling that I have been stung by a bee for no apparent reason at all.

Bees straddle the line between what is known about them and what still appears as simply miraculous. Honeybees can see flowers in the ultraviolet spectrum. They dance to communicate the distance and direction of forage. Bees come in three different genders. Rudimentary questions such as "How do they find their way back to the hive?" and the more complicated "How did bee society evolve in the first place?" continue to inspire imagination and are the focus of ongoing research. Many of us have seen honeybee hives, but where do the bumblebees and other solitary bees live? Where are they during the winter storms? Where are they at night? I have seen the holes of the mason bees, and the borings of the large black carpenter bees, but the squash bees in particular intrigue me—they make their appearance each spring when the zucchinis begin to bloom, and then. . .? I have read that during the winter the pupae are somewhere nearby in the soil, but I have never seen one. It is almost more fun to imagine that they appear out of thin air, as if the opening of the first squash blossoms in May triggers a magic portal that lures them out of another dimension.

One of my favorite stories about bees dates to 1934 when two French scientists, zoologist and aeronautical engineer Antoine Magnan and mathematician and engineer André Sainte-Laguë, calculated that the bulkiness of bumblebees combined with their undersized wings should make it impossible for them to fly, and the very fact that they could fly was contrary to the laws of physics. I would share this when I worked as an educator in the Colorado Rockies and we spied a bumblebee going about its business in the thin mountain air. Even after I came across a contemporary science article that explained how they flew I remained entranced: an extra twist of the bee's wing at the end of each stroke creates a miniature vortex in the air, which enhances lift for the subsequent wing beat. All of this happens 230 times a second. While scientists can now study bee flight with super-slow motion video cameras, wind tunnels, and even miniature robotic bees, the answers to some questions invariably lead to others. One researcher placed bees into a portable pressure chamber and found that the same bee could fly at pressures equivalent to the altitude of Mount Everest as well as in conditions that simulated locations below sea level such as Death Valley. Why would a bee have such a range of ability? The scientist did not know.

I walk outside on a sunny day in May and close my eyes. Sounds of the human world blend with the natural world: a breeze through the palm tree, a truck driving down the street, a Red-Shouldered Hawk calling to its mate, a neighbor doing yard work while talking on his cell phone. Amidst all of this, the soft hum of the bees is there, evidence that nature continues, constant, alive, and wondrous. The bees are not the beginning nor the culmination. Trace the flight paths of the bees and you create a tapestry that connects and embraces all that is important.

When I listen closely, I can hear it . . . in the center of it all.

CHAPTER 4

Food Forest Follies

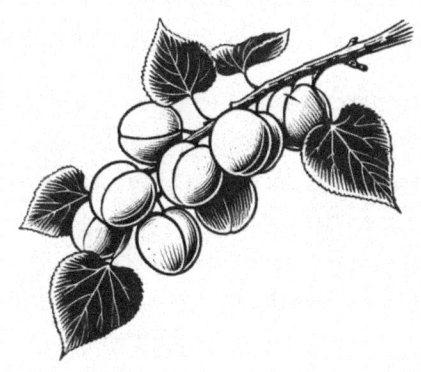

March of the Apricots

By some miracle of microclimates and sun angles, the neighbor's apricot tree over the back fence scoffs at the morning frost on the nearby rooftops and bursts out with soft pink blossoms at the end of February, a full two weeks before other apricot trees in my area. From there begins a gentle wave of valentine pink, gracefully migrating around the neighborhood. Eventually the blossoms emerge on the two trees in my own yard. I do not know what variety they are, but I don't think that it matters too much. I can say that all these trees are minimally maintained, partially ignored, and they all produce tasty fruit.

I leave it to the birds and squirrels to tell me when the 'cots over the back fence are ripe—the branches are too high for me to determine by the traditional "fruit fondle" technique. When partially-eaten apricots start falling, I know it is time to pull out my fruit picker, which is a small, clawed basket on the end of a yellow fiberglass telescoping pole. I am sure better tools exist as I must take care that the tines of the "claw" do not impale the fruit as I try to dislodge them from the limbs. But it works well enough. We eat the apricots fresh off the tree, chopped into oatmeal, or baked into crisps and other desserts, but pretty soon the apricot supply outpaces immediate demand. Our solution is to dry them, about 100 at a time. To preserve some of the color we soak them in orange juice first. They make for great holiday gifts and casual snacking throughout the year.

The second tree to ripen belongs to the next-door neighbors, a generally unkempt twiggy mess of branches that produces heavy and light crops of diminutive fruits in alternating years. I come out every four or five days to rescue the ones overhanging the sidewalk before they drop and add a layer of slimy orange sheen to the pavement below. After a couple of weeks, it is a losing battle. I become weary of lugging my ladder next door; the trees in my own yard are finally ripe, and they become the priority.

Tree number three yields the largest fruits, ones that actually might be worthy of a vendor's stall at the farmers' market. This is great, but now the problem is vacation: even the most devoted Chico resident needs to escape the summer heat for a few days, so my wife sends out a social media blast to friends and neighbors inviting them to pick the fruit. I always wish for our gleaner friends to be more ambitious, but I guess everyone is being polite to make sure enough fruit remains for the next person. We return to find dozens of pulpy deposits beneath the tree.

By the time the fruit comes ripe on our other tree, we are rather sick of apricots. The tree itself is a gnarled, diseased mess dappled with hard marble-sized amber globes of sap. Every year I fear that it may be the tree's last. Consequently, I don't invest too much time in caring for it, so each year it looks a bit more scraggly and produces smaller and smaller fruit. But it does produce. The scrub jays, which denied us the first apricots of the season just a few weeks prior, are now useless in consuming their share; perhaps they are also seeking a more varied diet. This is the time when bags of apricots start mysteriously appearing on our neighbors' door knobs. Meanwhile, the rest of the fruits falls to the ground and merges with the wood chips below, and the whole mess bakes in the sun to become a massive cellulose granola bar that is appreciated mostly by fruit flies.

Dr. Frankenstein's Grapefruit Failure

It took me over 40 years before I acquired a taste for grapefruits. My father had always been a big fan. On a typical morning, I could find him deftly handling that special curved grapefruit knife, separating the fruit from the peel as he read the morning newspaper. Grapefruits, however, were not designed for youngsters, and other than the occasional grapefruit-flavored soda at a fancy party, I didn't like its sour-bitter tang. I got more adventurous after moving to Chico, occasionally purchasing a couple of fruits at the farmers' market. The pink blush, juiciness, and hint of sweetness earned it my respect—you could say we became friendly acquaintances—but we were far from bosom buddies (unlike, say, white nectarines).

Once in a while, I would sample a grapefruit overhanging an alley fence, and more often than not I would be disappointed, if not outright disgusted, with the outcome. And then the day came when I discovered what would turn out to be the nonpareil of all grapefruit trees, growing just around the corner from my home.

This particular tree had long ago merged with an adjacent dilapidated fence and an out-of-control wisteria, which is the main reason why it had taken me so long to notice it. It was difficult to tell what was supporting what. The tree itself was a disheveled mess of branches and twigs interspersed with an assortment of green fruit, ripe fruit, overripe fruit, and rotten balls of moldy, grapefruit mush. Much of the tree was overhanging the sidewalk, and I picked two fruits that afternoon, juiced them, and then immediately went back for more. The sour-bitter grapefruit taste was there, but it was blended perfectly with a type of sweetness normally reserved for a Valencia orange. The result was addictive. The juice was like a zippy song with a catchy beat: you don't want it to end, you just want to indulge in the experience of it saturating the taste buds on your tongue and the back of your throat for as long as possible.

My family enjoyed the fruits from that tree for three years until I biked past one morning and found all of the branches had been sawed off and piled unceremoniously on the side of the street. The owners had decided that a new fence was worth more to them than an old citrus tree.

I was told the tree had been cut down the previous afternoon. The leaves were still green; the fruit was still there. I gathered up as many grapefruits as I could easily reach, then I levered up a branch and mined for more among the thicket of downed limbs. I biked away with about 100 pounds of fruit in my bike trailer. There were far too many for my family to eat, so I shared as much as I could. I was overcome with enormous sadness—these were the last fruits; there would be no more. This was the tree that had taught me a deep appreciation for grapefruits. My gastronomical spirit was indebted to this plant! There must be something I could do! Then the mad horticulturist in me emerged. I would graft! I would take clippings of the downed tree and splice them onto the orange and lemon trees in my yard! Yes! Certainly, I was aware that the odds of success were not high: the leaves on the grapefruit were already going limp, I had no experience with grafting, and it was probably the wrong season (is there a grafting season for citrus trees?)—but hey, I had a pair of clippers, a pocket knife, a roll of plastic stretchy green arborist ribbon, and an internet connection. One thing was certain: if I didn't try it, there was no way I would ever enjoy those grapefruit again.

I snipped off ten pencil-thick clippings, biked them home, and quickly dunked them in a bucket of water. I gave myself a fifteen-minute YouTube education on grafting citrus, and off I went, a freshly minted tree surgeon. With my pocketknife, I made V-shaped cuts in the grapefruit limbs and matched them to chisel-shaped cuts on the lemon and orange trees. Finally, I secured everything as tightly as I could with tape. Then there was nothing left to do but eat the grapefruit that I had picked and wait.

A year later I sadly removed ten desiccated twigs that were hanging from my trees. My attempts at grapefruit tree resurrection had failed. So long, dearest grapefruit tree. May I someday meet another with fruit just as sweet. 'Tis better to have grafted and lost than never to have grafted at all.

Nightmare on Avocado Street

As a native Californian, there is a part of me that feels the weekly, if not daily, enjoyment of avocados is my birthright. California grows 95% of the avocados in the United States and is the third largest producer of avocados worldwide, second only to Mexico and Brazil. But despite being among such a bounty, avocado addiction is costly, with each piece of fruit running a dollar or more. The solution to this economic dilemma was obvious, and, according to numerous sources, delightfully simple. With three toothpicks, a jar of water, an avocado pit, and a sunny window sill, I could grow my own tree. But I am not a selfish person; everybody deserves an avocado tree! My slogan would be a sapling in every garden pot, and I set out to become the Johnny Appleseed of avocados. Little did I know I would instead become the Dr. Moreau of the horticultural world.

Avocado trees are subtropical in origin and have a preference for the moderate temperatures of the Southern California coastal region. This is why 98% of all commercial avocado production in California takes place in San Diego, Riverside, Ventura, and Santa Barbara Counties. In contrast, my home of Chico has an annual temperature variation of 80F degrees or more, and a 40F-degree temperature swing over a 24-hour period is not uncommon. There is a reason why almond trees, and not avocados, grow feral in the North State. But I was not deterred; there was evidence all around that my task, though challenging, was not impossible, and this fueled my resolve. To start with, all the local nurseries sell avocado trees, touting "cold tolerant" varieties like "Zutano" and "Mexicola." Yes, those businesses could simply be out to dupe the naïve backyard weekend warrior (it wouldn't be the first time), but I had seen some of these trees with my own eyes! A three-story monster grows on the grounds of a bed and breakfast just 20 minutes away, it drips with beautiful purple fruits each October. I know of at least two "Bacon" varieties growing in south Chico, and a third lurks in an alley not four blocks from my house. And then there is the mystical, mythical "Duke" avocado, which was first propagated in Butte County in 1912. The skin of the fruit is light green and thin enough to eat, but they are also too delicate to withstand being crated and transported to market without bruising, which is apparently the reason why they were never widely cultivated. The Duke is said to originate from near Monterrey, Mexico, though avocado historians who have since scoured the region have failed to locate any such source trees. A small grove of the trees still stands resilient on a family farm at the base of Table Mountain near Oroville, California. They had a stand at the farmers' market, I purchased about two dozen fruits.

The mission began well enough. My modest greenhouse consisted of two sunny windows where there was enough room to start 20 pits in jars of tap water. Of these, a more than respectable 70% sprouted, and after about a year I transplanted them to one-gallon pots. As further insurance towards future guacamole grandeur, I also purchased two "established" avocado saplings from a local nursery, in hopes of cutting a year or two off the seven years it reportedly takes for a tree to mature enough to produce fruit.

Things quickly began to go awry. By decree of Murphy's Law, my most expensive investments—the saplings—were the first to perish. One acted as if being transplanted into my yard was the equivalent of being dipped in acid. A week after being placed in the ground, the leaves wilted and turned brown. I tried dripping some "Superthrive: World Champion Activator, Transplanter, Extra Grower, Perfector" to the base of the trunk. The dark green snake-oil liquid did none of these things for the plant.

The other sapling did a bit better and survived its first summer but then went the way of the tomato plants one frigid December morning when it decided its destiny was being an annual rather than a perennial—minus the part about producing seeds that would sprout the following season. By the end of February, I finally decided its brown, desiccated form was causing the rest of the yard to be depressed, so I dug it up, roots and all, only to find a viable sprout emerging from the base of the trunk. Or at least it had been viable right up until the moment that I jammed my shovel into its roots. Now it was a shredded mess, and it became the second sapling to enrich the compost bin.

Meanwhile, the plants in one-gallon pots remained on the sunny side of the house, shielded from the horrors that were occurring in the backyard. Sadly, they didn't fare very well either. The leaves on one seemed to suddenly mottle and then detach. Another pot somehow caught too much sun and not enough rain, and the sapling within did not appreciate being anchored in the resulting cement-like dirt clod. A few I gave away—these were the lucky ones—sent off as refugee shrubs in hopes they would reach more fertile ground. Eventually I was down to just two. The first I planted in a "protected" corner of the yard, a spot near the house that I hoped would have its own avocado-favorable microclimate. The second one I moved into a ten-gallon pot, and it spent the next year and half migrating between the deck and sunny indoor space near the kitchen. After the 40-pound potted tree made its third such journey, my back told me it was time for that plant, too, to find a permanent home in the yard. That same year an outdoor project forced the displacement of the first tree; I transplanted it to what I hoped would be an equally sheltered location beneath the canopy of an overhanging mulberry. No such luck. Gophers discovered the young roots and subsequently turned them into a dinner salad. The other sapling succumbed to what proved to be a comparatively mild Chico winter.

So that was it. I was defeated, but to justify my failures I developed a theory that all of Butte County's avocado trees must have been planted during a Northern California focused, 20-year global warming event that took place between 1960 and 1980. But even this fantasy was dispelled when I came across a healthy five-year-old sapling in southwest Chico. Its leaves fluttered as I strolled past, mocking me, rubbing salt into the wound, salt that I would rather be sprinkling into guacamole. I was finally ready to hang up my mad scientist lab coat when my inquisitive three-year-old daughter became fascinated with an avocado pit. And I couldn't help myself. I pulled out a jar and the box of toothpicks and went back to work.

Had the cycle of futility begun anew? Perhaps. But the following spring, rather than uproot the twiggy carcasses of my final two casualties, I trimmed them down to the ground. There, at the base of both plants, a hint of lime green stem was visible just below the decrepit brown. Upon closer inspection I saw small red buds swelling, preparing to emerge through the burr clover and crabgrass that I call the lawn. I think a seven-year timeline for making guacamole from backyard fruits might be a tad bit ambitious, but I am prepared to play the long game, telling myself, year after year, that it will be worth it.

Neighborly Oranges

The slow cooker recipe called for a ½ cup of orange juice. We used to keep a container of Trader Joe's concentrated frozen orange juice on hand, but they stopped carrying it years ago. Then I spied the orange tree across the street. The previous owners had moved out a few months before, and they had been fine with us retrieving a few fruits every now and again. I had been warned that they were not very good. I recalled juicing some a couple years back, and at the time I found the juice to be palatable if a bit sour and watery.

Orange juice, reconstituted from cardboard canisters of frozen slush, was once my drink of choice. It was what I had growing up as a child ("Part of this nutritious breakfast!"), and it was what I drank in college. My roommates said I had orange juice coursing through my veins. Once, when I was about 9, my family visited my grandparents in south Florida. The orange juice at the restaurant was foreign, odd, and I didn't like it. It was fresh-squeezed.

I eventually learned that orange juice has a lot of sugar (yes, I know it is "natural sugar," but it is still sugar), and my body really didn't need (or shouldn't have) a quart of orange juice every couple of days. I also learned that the oranges in my area are a winter fruit that usually reach peak sweetness around January-February. And lastly, I have, over the years, come to the conclusion that sweet, locally-grown oranges are a delicious treat best savored when in season and not a constitutional right to be able to access 365 days a year.

Back to the present. It was mid-August. We had experienced heat wave after heat wave since the end of May, and there had not been a drop of rain for about as long. The sun was barely visible through the smoky haze of the most recent wildfire in the nearby mountains, and a fine dusting of ash was everywhere. I again gazed out the window—yes, there were oranges on the tree, but they had been dangling there for over five months, including the past few weeks of 90F+ degree weather. I figured it was likely that each orange would yield as much liquid as a dry sponge with a hint of wood smoke flavoring. But perhaps, just perhaps, I might be able to extract enough moisture to reach my half cup quota. It wasn't like I was hosting a brunch where the guests might take a hearty swig only to abruptly expel a sour, ash-flavored spray of orange beverage across the table. I was just going to dump the juice into a crockpot.

I had met the new neighbors just once, and it was too early in the morning to give them a courtesy knock on the door. The tree was on the far side of the garage away from the front windows. With air quality so poor, few people were out. I needed the juice now. Slow cooker recipes need to get started early, and I didn't have time to wait for the neighbors to wake up. I started playing the "Mission Impossible" soundtrack in my head, grabbed a cloth bag, put on my loafers, and hoofed it across the street. I allowed myself 45 seconds to pick some fruit and then skedaddled, undetected. Tom Cruise's Ethan Hunt (or if you prefer, Peter Graves's James Phelps) would have been proud.

I had grabbed 11 oranges. I rinsed off the ash and sliced the first one in half, expecting the worst. But somehow, it looked, and smelled, like an orange. I juiced three, poured myself a jigger's worth, and took a tentative sip. A bit warm, but delicious. I was pleasantly shocked. I juiced the rest, added the appropriate amount to the crockpot, and shared the remainder—a couple of cups—with my family.

I think it's time to say hi to the new neighbors again.

Peach Pit Conspiracy

One September, a remarkable variety of peach appeared at the farmers' market. A firm, medium-sized fruit, it had fuzzy, blood-red skin with hints of dark green and orange. The flesh inside was crimson near the pit and cream-colored near the surface. The flavor, while not the five-star deliciousness of a midsummer peach, was still delightful, made more so since the five-star fruits were no longer available. And best of all, the vendor informed me that I could plant the pit and get a tree that will produce the same fruit. She called it an "Indian Peach."

At first, I was amazed that this could be possible. Didn't all modern fruit trees come from grafted saplings purchased from the local nursery? Could I really grow a perfectly fine tree for the cost of a single piece of fruit? Had I been a hapless victim of brainwashing by that devious horticultural industry? Various internet sources give differing answers (as they are prone to do). Naysayers make it sound like such an endeavor is likely doomed to failure and could very well bring on the apocalypse, stating that you might wait a decade or more only to find out that your tree is intolerant of the weather in your area, or is especially prone to disease, or produces bitter fruit, undersized fruit, or perhaps no fruit at all. The Penn State College of Agricultural Sciences puts it bluntly:

> *The new plant will be the same kind of plant, but its fruit and vegetative portions may not look the same as the parent . . .. Therefore, all fruit trees must be vegetatively propagated by either grafting or budding methods.*

However, other sources said "Go for it!" with the disclaimer that your level of success depends on a number of factors including the variety of fruit and whether your seed or pit contains genetic material from nearby fruit trees. Apples and pears are generally not recommended. (Their sexual biology—which I won't delve into here—makes the likelihood of achieving a tasty outcome pretty unlikely.) Some research should also go into your growing conditions. Just because I can purchase dates at the Chico farmers' market doesn't mean I can grow a fruiting date palm in my backyard.[1] However, peach, nectarine, and apricot pits frequently get a thumbs up, and I read that they can yield pie-worthy fruit-bearing trees in four years or less.

Gardeners like myself hear what they want to hear, so I disregarded the scare tactics of the agricultural academics and planted five Indian peach pits in the backyard. The Indian peach, it turns out, might be one of the best varieties to try growing from a pit. As early as 1562, this kind of peach was introduced to the Americas by early explorers of the Gulf Coast. The tree, aided by Native Americans, slowly naturalized up and down the Atlantic seaboard. Colonist William Penn observed wild Indian peaches as far north as Philadelphia in 1683. (Take that, Penn State.) The tree also made its way south. In his book *1491*, Charles C. Mann notes that by 1836 peach trees were the main source of firewood for the city of Buenos Aires. The Indian peach is patriotic too: Thomas Jefferson selected it as one of 38 varieties of peaches growing in his orchards at Monticello.

Flash forward about 200 years to my yard in Chico where three of the five pits sprouted. Eighteen months later I chose my champion and carefully dug up the other two saplings and gave them away. The tree bore its first flowers at two years and yielded a dozen peaches after three. They were, as promised by the vendor, identical to the parent fruit. The first bumper crop came at year four, and I also noted that the tree seemed more resistant to

---

1. There are two fruiting date palms in downtown Chico of unknown heritage. The dates are palatable, but nothing to write home about.

peach leaf curl than some of the other fruit trees in the yard. Year five was looking just as promising, with deep pink blossoms giving way to dozens of fruits, until disaster struck during the third week of April. The unripe fruits shriveled, the leaves withered, and soon all I had was kindling, worthy only of a fireplace in Buenos Aires.

A conversation at a potluck meandered into tomato territory. A new friend had read a couple of my previously published articles, and somehow arrived at the strange conclusion that I knew something about gardening. He described in detail his tomato woes from the previous summer, when his sungold plants missed a key memo, and ended up with orange-yellow leaves instead of orange-yellow tomatoes. The whole plant expired a few days later. "This didn't happen to me last year. What do you think?"

What did I think? I pondered this for a brief moment, flashing through a decade of gardening failures and successes and multiple essays in which I provide creative reasons for both outcomes. Then I looked him in the eye and said: "Sometimes things just die. All the more reason to appreciate what lives."

Plum Tree Resurrection

We never asked the previous owners why the magnolia tree needed to be removed, but we should have. When my wife and I started planting our "home orchard" (read: devious marketing term created by the bareroot fruit tree industry), we naively whacked away at old roots to dig the holes for our 3 apple trees, 3 pear trees, 2 plum trees, 4 pluot trees, and the aforementioned Indian peach. Later that fall, clusters of mushrooms emerged—densely packed brown ones—at the base of two of the trees. They looked cute at the time, but over the next ten years, the trees died off while the mushrooms kept coming back and spreading through the soil from tree to tree.

I attempted multiple methods of killing the mushroom, but nothing worked. I even tried cooking and eating it, which was a mistake. (I spent much of that night asking the porcelain gods to forgive my foolishness).[2] The fungus couldn't take full credit for every tree that died. Aphids played

---

2. If you must know, the mushroom was *Armillaria mellea*, which some (but not all) mycophiles consider to be edible.

the role of accomplices, as did fire blight (a bacterial disease), which did in the apples and pears. Eventually, our orchard resembled the end of *The Lorax* but with no truffula seeds left to plant. Until . . .

Two years ago, a scraggly twig grew from the base of one of the stumps, eventually reaching a height of two feet. Last year it got to four feet, flowered, and produced a single delicious plum. Whether the growth emerged from above the original graft or below I do not know. But I don't care. Perhaps it is just a matter of time before the mushroom comes back, but in the meantime, live long and prosper, little plum.

Conserving Seeds

"Dad, can you get mandarin oranges at the farmers' market this week?"

"But we have a mandarin tree in the back yard. It needs to be picked; the fruit is really sweet."

"Yes, but our mandarins have seeds."

And she's right, of course. Our mandarins do have seeds. Lots of seeds. Fifteen to twenty per fruit (and the fruits ain't that big). Whenever I eat one of our mandarins, I feel like a baseball manager spitting out three innings worth of seeds. My theory is this: once there were seeds in all seedless mandarins, and they had to go somewhere. Well, they went to our yard. To our fruits. I call it "The Law of Conservation of Mandarin Seeds." So, when you wolf down your next seedless mandarin orange, think of us.

You're welcome.

Avocado Epilogue

You may be asking, whatever became of my mission to grow a Duke avocado? For those that don't know, the cultivation of the Duke is Butte County's contribution to the avocado world (it's true, you can look it up). This question becomes especially more relevant now that Chaffin Family Orchards, my favorite avocado source, is no longer selling produce at the farmers' market. The Miocene Canal, a key source of their water, was damaged during the 2018 Camp Fire and will not be repaired, so they have been forced to change the focus of their operations.

To add insult to injury, I can't for certain recall which pits I planted were Dukes, and which were Bacons, also from a neighborhood tree. I CAN say—drum roll—that the tree lives! Its growth has been slow, but it is now a healthy-looking 11-year-old-tree about ten feet tall. Duke? Bacon? I have no idea. Its existence thus far has been that of a fruitless shrub. My guacamole has yet to be sourced from my backyard. I will be in touch in 2030.

Avocado Epilogue, Part 2

April, 2024: The first flowers appeared on the avocado tree! Not a single bud matured into an avocado, but hey, progress is progress!

CHAPTER 5

Food on the Go

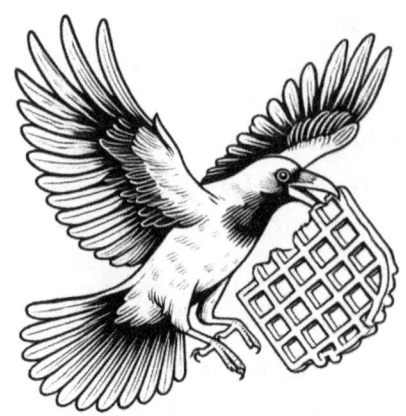

A Survival Guide to the Rental House Kitchen

When you arrive at your rental, go on a scavenger hunt to find the kitchen "ten essentials." In no particular order: 1) salt, 2) olive oil, 3) a roll of paper towels, 4) a metal spatula, 5) a can opener, 6) the largest mug, 7) a pot with a matching lid, 8) a scouring pad, 9) towels to dry the dishes, 10) the "Popcorn" button on the microwave. This last item is the most important. If you know nothing else about how to operate the appliances in your rental, this simple button will be what saves you from starvation. Need some hot water for tea? Press "Popcorn" and then "Start." Reheat last night's Mexican take-out? Same thing. Even though the setting might have a three-minute run, you can still shut it off halfway through. Don't bother with any of the other buttons, this will lead you to frustration, and frustration leads to the Dark Side. Note: Do NOT under any circumstances actually try to make some popcorn. It's a trap—that's what they want you to do, and it is a recipe for disaster and will likely result in setting off the smoke alarm.

Be advised: the knives in the rental will always be dull. Unless you packed a pocket knife, there is nothing you can do about it. Large pots can double as serving bowls. Avoid the beat-up Teflon pans; I promise you that a stainless steel or an iron skillet will be there, hidden in a dark corner of the lower cupboard. Iron is an essential mineral; 20-year-old Teflon flakes are not.

Don't get frustrated when you can't find a matching lid to a plastic Tupperware storage container. Those containers are probably too gross to touch your food anyway. Instead, find the cabinet with the plates and bowls. Any self-respecting rental house will have no fewer than five sizes of mismatched thrift store Corelle bowls and plates that, when used in tandem (plate over bowl, or bowl flipped over plate), will do a fine job of storing your leftovers.

If you come across a container of *Tajin* seasoning, you are in luck. *Tajin* is the Elvish waybread of the spice cabinet. In a pinch, it will keep your meals from being boring and drab, and serve as a substitute for salsa, tabasco sauce, and most dried or powdered Latin American and Italian spices.

Finally, don't be tempted to sample from the tub of discount ice cream a previous tenant left in the freezer, the one looks like it came from the Siberian permafrost. That's just disgusting.

Air Travel Provisions

Our carry-on luggage is a traveling food pantry. It is worth it, however, to fend off hunger and grumpiness as we wait in the terminal, or in a line to retrieve a rental car, or sit in a crowded plane that is motionless on the tarmac for no apparent reason. And we really don't like forking out $15 for a mediocre chopped chicken salad from one of the airport dining establishments. So our carry-ons are loaded, and we are not just talking granola bars. We pack as if we expect to be stranded by a freak, once-in-a millennia hurricane, even if we are in a city that has never experienced a hurricane.

Our travel rations have raised the eyebrows of many TSA employees, but they have never kept us from making our flight. They are as follows: Sliced apples or nectarines, five hard boiled eggs (pre-salted), sautéed Brussel sprouts (the round shape is convenient), sliced salami, a medley of cut cucumber, carrots, and sweet peppers, pluots or mandarin oranges (depending on the season), leftover meatballs, and yes, mixed nuts. All are packed neatly in plastic or metal travel containers (one-quart yogurt containers are my go-to), and are sealed with masking tape and labeled with a sharpie as needed.

Of course, despite these efforts, at least one of my daughters invariably notices the resident food court Chipotle during our layover, and I still find myself queuing up in the food line and forking over $25 for two underwhelming burrito bowls. Thwarted. I guess Brussel sprouts and salami slices aren't everyone's cup of tea.

Spaghetters

"It looks like we made too much pasta."

We were seven miles from the trailhead, on a large granite sheet overlooking the Kern River in the southern Sierra. We had just concluded a very satisfying meal, but indeed, about three cups worth of poorly strained angel hair still sat in the bottom of the pot. Angel hair pasta is a great backpacking choice because it cooks fast.[1] However, it is also hard to eyeball dry pasta and make a prediction as to how many servings it will yield and how hungry everyone is going to be.

As serious "leave no trace" hikers, we were in a quandary: we weren't going to bury the food, and we hadn't made a campfire to burn it. Adding additional intrigue to our few options was that we had already realized that there were no tall trees nearby suitable for hanging our remaining food stuffs (breakfast, lunch, and snacks for the next day). Since we were lacking a bear canister as well, we had made the rather unorthodox decision to tie a rope to a nearby sapling and then let the food dangle 15 feet down against the granite cliff, and 30 feet above the boulder-strewn river, and hope for the best. In the end, we put the lid on the pot of pasta, tied the rope to the handle, and dangled that too.

Morning came without incident—no bears, raccoons, or other varmints discovered our food bags or the pot. However, the pasta was still there needing to be dealt with. We had no desire to pack it out, and besides, we wanted to use the pot to boil some water for oatmeal.

The angel hair had congealed in the bottom of the pot and looked like a mess of blonde worms. Luckily, we had butter.

---

1. I have since discovered that the Asian-style "mei fun" noodles cook even faster: just two to four minutes in boiling water.

My two hiking companions watched warily as I fired up the stove and melted a generous chunk of butter in the skillet. I cut the pasta mass into quarters, and carefully transferred them to the pan, sautéing them to a golden brown.

We called them "spaghetters." They were quite good.

Unexpected Rhubarb

My family went for a stroll along a dirt Forest Service road near Butte Meadows. The scenery at 5,000 feet is one of mountains and fir and pine trees, creeks and meadows, summer wildflowers, and, about a mile from the parking lot, one stalwart rhubarb plant. This was not the native Indian rhubarb, but rather was the species known to European immigrants, the one where the stems are chopped and then combined with sugar and strawberries and baked into a pie. This lone plant was growing in the middle of an open gravelly meadow with a creek flowing about 50 yards away. It was large, maybe three feet in diameter and just as high, and it was in bloom, with dozens of insects swarming and crawling over its tightly-packed cream-colored flowers.

I tried to imagine its history. It is not a stretch to envision that there was once a homestead, or at least a cabin nearby, with sheep grazing the meadow. Early pioneer wives often brought dormant rhubarb roots with them to plant, so it is possible that the specimen in the meadow could be decades old. Little else hints of a cabin site. There are no remains of a chimney or a foundation—just some rusted bits of metal, some broken pottery, and that's about it. This was not the first time I had stumbled across similar plants that were proof of pioneer homes that disappeared years before. I can recall walks through the woods where I had encountered spindly lilac shrubs, sprawling rose bushes, isolated outposts of daffodils, and even the occasional apple tree, all still homesteading of their own accord.

I briefly considered separating some of the rhubarb root and trying to get this living bit of local history established in a corner of my garden, but I read that rhubarb doesn't tend to be heat tolerant, so it likely wouldn't do well trying to survive a Chico summer. I allowed myself to be satisfied with leaving it in peace. Hopefully it will continue to stir the imagination of others in the decades to come.

Mountain Air

Certainly there is truth to the opinion that "everything tastes better in the backcountry." Indeed, but it can also be stated that some meals do taste a lot better than others. It took me two decades to figure this out. I have since learned that there is a fine art to finding that sweet spot between minimizing weight, maximizing convenience, and maintaining a high standard of gastronomical acceptability for one's backcountry repasts.

In my experience, there are several backpacking food manufacturers that believe customers are most concerned about weight and convenience while at the same time maximizing shelf life. Food is freeze-dried or powdered (or both) and then vacuum-packed into the smallest volume possible. What is lost in natural flavor and hue is replaced by chemicals—the usual mixture of salts, preservatives, and colors. The end result are meals that are lightweight, quick to prepare, and, in my experience, generally mediocre in taste and lead to high country flatulence of the greatest degree, providing a whole new dimension to the concept of "a mountain breeze."

During my Boy Scout years, I tolerated "Western Omelette" that, prior to cooking, included what looked like regurgitated chunks of dehydrated tomatoes, onions, and peppers mixed into a yellowish egg-dust; vacuum-packed "Beef Stroganoff," "Pasta Primavera" and "Minestrone Soup" (as scouts we always asked the question, "Soup strewn with mines?"); and also hummus powder, mashed potato powder, and banana pudding powder. At the time, I simply didn't know any better.

Many of the meals were much more appreciated for their entertainment value than for their culinary enjoyment. One backpacking food company produced a lunch kit that included dense round biscuits, a meat-spread, and a hard candy product. The spreads came in three flavors—chicken, ham, and tuna—but they all looked the same, kind of like cat food (they were even packaged in small Fancy Feast-like tins). The hard candies were comparable to Starburst fruit chews without the chewiness and were tough enough to dislodge a molar or survive a nuclear apocalypse. But the real sport was found in the biscuits, which resembled bulked-up versions of Ritz crackers. Old-timers used to call them "hardtack" or "pilot biscuits," but for 14-year-old Boy Scouts, they were much more serviceable as projectile weapons, like ninja stars without the bladed points (but still nearly as lethal).

Later I learned the contents of the "backpacking food" packages can easily be replicated at home for less cost, with less artificial chemicals, more flavor, and the same amount of weight. Rice is rice, pasta is pasta, oatmeal is oatmeal, granola is granola. I now dry some of my garden or farmers' market vegetables in the food dehydrator a few days in advance of each trip, and reconstitute zucchini, tomatoes, onions, and peppers in the same pot where I boil my pad thai noodles. My excursions also now tend to be shorter in duration, so I splurge and include some fresh produce now and again. My favorite is the Armenian cucumber, which compliments crackers, slices of dry salami, and smoked gouda cheese as part of a perfect creek-side lunch. Armenian cucumbers (technically a type of melon) are hardy enough to survive being packed into a bear canister for a long weekend.

My go-to hiking nosh involves reaching into a gallon-size Ziplock bag and grabbing a handful of raisins and dry-roasted peanuts, mixed 50-50. Sure, go ahead and add your M&Ms, or coconut flakes, or pumpkin seeds or date chunks if it makes you happy. But know that it isn't necessary—everything tastes good in the backcountry. And besides, the simplicity of "good old raisins and peanuts" allows you to call it by its proper name, "Gorp." But you probably already knew that.

Waffle Toss Champion

"Firing up Little Moe!"

Little Moe was the name which my roommate, John, and I had given to the smaller of our two waffle irons during our senior year of college. (Its larger cousin was Big Red.) Waffles were our morning sustenance that year. We're not talking Eggos here—this was the real deal. We kept a quart of homemade waffle batter in the fridge at the ready, and our kitchen was stocked with "I Can't Believe It's Not Butter" purchased by the discount bulk tubfull along with a gallon jug of Mrs. Butterworth's. (Looking back, I can't believe I bought I Can't Believe It's Not Butter . . .). While we never ditched the butter substitute that year, fortunately John came home from a spring break visit to New England with a two-quart jar full of maple syrup. The penciled cursive writing on the masking tape label read, simply, "Vermont Pure." That was the day we bid farewell to Mrs. Butterworth's.

We would invite a small group of friends to join us for waffles, at least once a week, plugging in both Big Red and Little Moe. Dining time varied based on our class schedules; we tried to mix it up so that everyone could participate. What didn't change was the traditional closing of the meal—the famous Waffle Toss. After we all were done eating, we would cook up one last batch of waffles a little extra crispy—dark brown, but not quite burnt. We would then gather up our school gear and the extra-hard waffles and walk the two blocks to campus, where we would pause on the manicured shore of Lakum Duckum (pronounced "lake-uhm duck-uhm"). Lakum Duckum is a human-made pond along College Creek, which forms a natural boundary between the college academic buildings and a number of student residence halls. In the 1920s, the creek is said to have supported a chinook salmon run. Today it supports mallards and goldfish.

The Waffle Toss rules were simple—you got one chance to fling your 4 x 4-inch waffle as far across Lakum Duckum as possible. The person with the longest toss was crowned the reigning Waffle Toss Champion and earned bragging rights as well as the honor of throwing first the following week. In truth, the real winners were always the ducks, who enjoyed cleaning up after competitions. A 50-foot throw would allow your waffle to reach the far shore, but there were obstacles. Toss it too high and overhanging tree branches sent your waffle plunging down into the middle of the pond. Boulders also impeded heaves that flew too low. Furthermore, we found that waffles were not really the most aerodynamic of objects, and they had a tendency to twist and dive unexpectedly in flight.

The ideal target was a patch of lawn on the far side of the creek, between two large shrubs. If you were lucky, a spinning waffle would bounce and roll up the embankment, adding distance. Waffles were tossed backhanded, like a frisbee, or overhead, like a boomerang. I usually chose the latter.

The most memorable toss came in the late spring. My rapidly-rotating throw dove below the branches, bypassed the boulders, and hit high on the far bank. Still spinning, it bounced twice, cleared the lawn, shot the gap between the shrubs, and hopped the curb, ending up two feet into the street on the other side. It was only there for a few seconds. At that point a crow swooped down, grabbed the waffle in its talons, and took off. Our jaws dropped, and the whooping began. In that moment, I became the reigning Waffle Toss Champion. Forever. I like to imagine that waffle is still flying, perpetually airborne over the fields and foothills of Eastern Washington and beyond.

The Banana Boat: Queen of the Camping Desserts

When a s'more dreams, it dreams it's a banana boat.

1. Take an unpeeled banana and place it in the middle of a 12 x 12-inch-square piece of heavy-duty aluminum foil.

2. Carefully slice the banana lengthwise, as you would for a banana split. If possible, don't slice completely through, but try to leave the bottom part of the peel intact.

3. Open the banana like a book. Along the length of the banana, insert four or five pieces of chocolate (or a handful of chocolate chips) and four half-pieces of marshmallow. Optional: Insert crumbled graham cracker or berries.

4. Gently fold the banana back together and securely wrap it with aluminum foil, carefully creasing the edges of the foil to reduce leakage.

5. Place the package in the warm coals of a campfire for 7-10 minutes.

6. Use sticks or long barbeque tongs to remove the package from the coals. Allow to cool for ten minutes.

7. Carefully unwrap the foil. Eat with a spoon.

October 7, 2005

"Hunger forces us to stop at 'The Country Kitchen' in Princeton, Illinois, at around 8 p.m. A poor choice. Amy manages to stomach, somehow, a defrosted, flattened, salmon-parts burger, lightly grilled and placed on a bed

of shredded iceberg lettuce. My food is the same, but with chicken. It tastes like it looks—forgettable, though in reality we will never forget that this was a pretty awful meal. Amy makes me promise that we will never eat such food again and that we will never let our future children eat such food. I agree, and we drive on."

CHAPTER 6

The Witch Doctor's Pantry

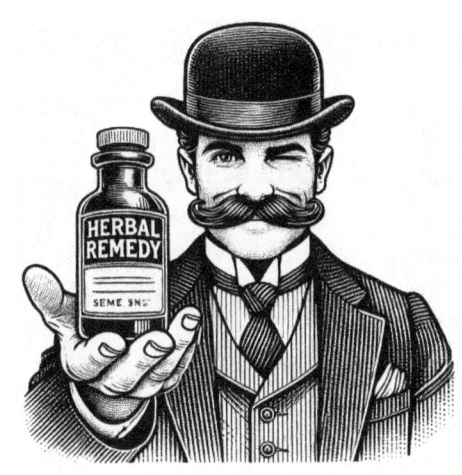

Do you have foot odor? Back pain? Seasonal allergies? Are you seeking relief from winter sniffles? Does your pee stink?

Madams and gentlemen, gather 'round, don't be shy! A cure for everything lies within! No reason to make an unnecessary trip to the drug store, just open up your pantry! Why call the doctor when the most esteemed experts of the world are available on your smartphone screen, just a few taps away?

Grab the sea salt, the cayenne powder, a couple of choice weeds from the backyard, and ignore that dusty bottle of snake oil over there—it's expired. I have a menagerie of much more modern remedies to remove your aches and pains. Massage the right food onto your body, and you will be healed!

For better (or for worse) my family has tried every concoction, every salve, and every tea so you don't have to. Unless, of course, you really want to . . .

Horehound

I had a sore throat. It was inevitable—the bug was going around the summer camp, and fellow staff members were feeling run-down and were hacking up green phlegm. At the time, I was really interested in identifying wild, edible, and useful plants using books from the camp's small natural history library. One field guide singled out horehound as the best remedy for a sore throat; luckily it was growing in abundance a short walk from my cabin.

Horehound is a weed that tastes pretty much the same way it sounds—really, really, really bitter. You can think of horehound as the bastard cousin of spearmint, and, despite its flavor, it has similar medicinal properties that are said to be helpful in relieving the symptoms of upper respiratory ailments. You used to be able to buy horehound candy at the old-timey drugstore, but now you can purchase a six-ounce package through new-timey Amazon, with delivery by Wednesday if you order it in the next six hours.

The guidebook gave a simple recipe for making an elixir by steeping horehound leaves in water and then mixing the resulting tea with honey. I found out that this is a great way to make honey taste really, really bad. It's hard to treat an illness if you can't get the medicine past your tongue.

Garlic Toes

Sadly, I think athlete's foot runs in my family ("Dad Joke," I couldn't resist). But it's true. There are certain weeks during the year when my daughters' toes itch, the skin on their feet is peeling, and when they pull their socks off in the car, we need to roll down the windows, and fast. Yes, I have used over-the-counter antifungal creams on my own leather-skinned doggies, but my wife and I had reservations about sullying our daughters' feet with those same big-pharma ointments. The internet, of course, has an alternative DIY solution for everything, including a plethora of ideas for crafting natural remedies for athlete's foot. Numerous websites tout the antimicrobial, antibacterial, and antifungal properties of crushed fresh garlic (though not anti-vampiral, as fans of the film *The Lost Boys* will readily affirm). Other internet bloggerscribes attribute similar properties to coconut oil, which is also said to be soothing on the skin. Well, we had garlic in the fridge, and coconut oil on the shelf, so why not provide our children's footsies with the best of both worlds?

Fast forward: A salve made of coconut oil and mashed garlic makes a person's feet smell a bit like slightly putrid Thai food, and, as a bonus, it adds oil stains to one's socks. It's effectiveness at eliminating athlete's foot is questionable. Eventually the fungus did go away—perhaps it ate it's fill of dead skin and moved on, or maybe it simply died of laughter rather than from the so-called potent garlic toxins enhanced with oil of *Cocos nucifera*. It is also likely that the kids simply stopped mentioning their itching toes because they no longer wanted us to smear them with garlic-coconut slime. The remaining two tablespoons of unused mixture sat in a jar in the fridge for six months before being found in the back corner, at which time we added the contents to the compost bin.

Magic Powder

I made an appointment to see a local witch doctor because I had an ache in my hip that wouldn't go away. The practitioner's name is actually Daniel, but I use the term "witch doctor" because, quite simply, I don't know exactly how he does what he does, but I do know that most of the time, whatever he does, it works. I lie on my back, tell him what hurts, and then he pokes and prods my abdomen for a bit. Then he says "Let's try some proprioception."

I do my best to repeat the word. "Pope's conception?"

Daniel says it again, but it remains a tongue twister to me—one of those in-one-ear then garbled-in-the-brain sort of terms. According to the good people at Webmd.com, proprioception is "the body's ability to sense movement, action, and location" and probably is a word which chiropractors use in daily conversation over coffee. To me it sounds like part of a mystical incantation that Gandalf might say to gain access to a secret passageway. Gandalf—I mean Daniel—then bends my legs a bit, tells me to push my knees sidewise against his hands a few times, and then he massages in some key spots. Thirty minutes later I am on my way, pain-free. So when he suggests that I might consider taking diatomaceous earth to help ease joint pain, I don't hesitate in purchasing a two-pound bag. If this enchanted white powder is as effective as his proprio-spellcasting, well, that's good enough for me.

Yes, I do know what diatomaceous earth is. It is a fine, odorless white powder made from the crushed, fossilized remains of single-celled, aquatic organisms called diatoms. Their cell walls consist of silica, the same chemical that makes up glass. Over a long period of time, diatoms accumulated in the bottoms of rivers, streams, lakes, and oceans. Today, the resulting diatomaceous earth is mined and used in a variety of applications, ranging from pool filters to non-toxic pesticides to toothpaste.

I had not, however, heard of plain "food grade" diatomaceous earth, but that's what the package said, so I gave it a go. I tried a tablespoon in water, and the first thing I noticed was that it didn't really dissolve. Rather, it made the water cloudy for a few minutes and eventually sank to the bottom, so I pretty much needed to stir and drink it right away. It tasted like it looked: like very fine, flavorless grit. I tried it in some orange juice and ended up with gritty orange juice. I couldn't bear the idea of sprinkling it in with some food, so I finally settled on mixing it with coffee and stirring in a bit of sugar in an effort to distract myself from the grittiness, albeit with minimal success.

After a year of drinking gritty coffee, my joints felt . . . well, they felt a year older than when I started.

I knew what had happened. I had the magic powder, but I had never learned the magic words! Though even if I had, I probably wouldn't have been able to pronounce them properly, and this might have done more harm than good.

Move Over, Ivermectin?

A recent study found that nigella seed, known to gardeners as "Love-in-a-Mist," contains a compound that has the potential to serve as a therapy for COVID-19. If true, then my property is the Holy Grail for ending the pandemic! We have nigella everywhere! But sadly, the fine print from the research article is far from definitive: ". . . therapy of *N. sativa* [nigella] may reduce the adverse effects of conventional medicines by helping to decrease their doses. However, more randomized controlled trials are required to confirm the potential beneficial effects of *N. sativa* to treat the patients with COVID-19." Additionally, I learned that the flowers in my garden are *Nigella damascena* and not *N. sativa*. In short, my yard will not be curing COVID anytime soon. Let me be clear: **NIGELLA SEEDS ARE NOT A CURE FOR CORONAVIRUS**. But as a consolation, I do have a good Moroccan chicken recipe that calls for nigella seeds.

Orange Stinky Super Pee

Ah yes, the superfoods. You know them well—they hang out together in the breakroom refrigerator at the Hall of Justice: blueberries, pomegranate, kale, organ meats, turmeric root, almonds, sunchokes, cider vinegar, and of course, spinach (remember Popeye?). You've probably heard many of the buzz-phrases that "explain" why they are super: low glycemic index, high in antioxidants, nutrient dense, enhanced immunity, they are colorful, etc.

For me, however, the key is not what the food is supposed to do, but how it does it. That is why I place beets and asparagus high on that pedestal of culinary awesomeness. These foods provide near immediate evidence that they are working—the proof is in the porcelain (the toilet). Let's start with red beets. They turn your pee from a boring light yellow to a sunset orange hue. I know this must be good, because when I have seen images of surgeons working inside the human body, there is nothing in there that is the color of sunset orange. That color is not supposed to be there! Which is why, I believe, beets are so important—they help remove from the body that which does not belong, making you healthier and more super.

Then there is asparagus, one of the few vegetables that is referred to by its scientific name, which I take as a sign that this spring green is simply too impressive to even have a "common" name. I believe that asparagus works in a similar manner as the beet; in this case, helping the body to evacuate pungent odors that simply shouldn't be inside of us. There may be some readers that have no idea what I am talking about. "My pee doesn't stink after eating asparagus!" Well, actually it does. What scientists have found is that everyone produces asparagusic acid after eating asparagus; it's just that not everyone has the ability to smell it. (Go ahead, fact-checkers, prove me wrong).

Of course, the most important reason to include beets and asparagus in your diet is because your mother told you to.

Nice Cabbages

Had I said that to my spouse, I would have likely had any and all marital privileges revoked for a month, including, but not limited to, goodbye kisses, endearing smiles, and any physical contact beyond my wife accidentally kicking me in her sleep. Yes, I had just placed large cabbage leaves onto her breasts—at her request—but this is not what you think. Just a few weeks into motherhood, things were not going well, and my lovely wife was hurting. Her breasts were tender and swollen, her nipples were raw, and her milk production was minimal. Our newborn was always crying, and I was miserable by association. We were one big, unhappy family.

In an effort to alleviate my wife's suffering and increase her milk supply, we tried everything that the various professionals recommended to us or that we randomly discovered on the internet: hot packs, cold packs, soothing baths, "Mother's Milk" tea, "Lactation Support" tea, fennel tea, fenugreek tea, fennel and fenugreek tea, breast pumps (manual and electric), steamed spiced placenta (no, I am not kidding), and the banned medication Domperidone. We sought out the support of no fewer than four different lactation consultants—a profession I hadn't even known existed until that time—who offered encouragement, massage, and advice, but none of them could take away the pain or increase milk production. Then I read about cabbage leaves.

From Healthline.com: "While it sounds weird, it seems to have some basis in science: Because of certain plant compounds found in cabbage, the leaves may have an anti-inflammatory effect on breast tissue when applied directly to your skin." So we tried it. With the greenery on her boobs, my wife looked a bit like an R-rated Carmen Miranda, or perhaps a vegan version of the mermaid Ariel, who had swapped her scallop-shell bikini top for a plant-based alternative. But cabbages didn't work for her either. We tried both green and red.

In the end, the ultimate remedies were time and perseverance. Our baby daughter was nourished in part from milk from mom, some from formula, and some from a friend and breast milk donor, Rachel, to whom we are eternally grateful. Three years later things went much easier with our second child. We were able to use our cabbage purchase to make coleslaw and sauerkraut, and everybody was much happier.

Coffee and Cayenne

This one actually seems to work. I have found there is something about spicy food that helps keep the cough and throat nasties at bay. An eighth teaspoon of powdered cayenne in a warm Cuppa Joe does it for me, especially when I still need to do the duty of waking up at 6 a.m. to make breakfasts and get the kids off to school. I forgo the sweetener—I don't want to risk giving the germs any sugary treats to help them out. I can also recommend mixing some spicy curry paste or powder (or both) into scrambled eggs. Chase it with a mug of chicken broth, infused with another pinch of cayenne. And get a good night's sleep, if you can.

Honey Tastes Good

Yes, honey does taste good. Go ahead and add some to your peppermint tea if that's what it takes. But beyond the "spoonful of sugar (honey) helps the medicine go down," I am not convinced that it actually, well, does anything. Case in point: Much has been written about eating local honey as a means to alleviate seasonal allergies. The idea here, as I understand it, is that chemicals from the local pollen find their way into the honey; thus, ingesting this honey helps to build up one's tolerance to the pollen. A friend recently told me he swears by it, but just a few days later another colleague asked the poignant question: How does one get the bees to actually go to the flowers that a person is allergic to? He also noted that people who have a seasonal allergy to walnut pollen or grass pollen—a.k.a. hay fever (like yours truly)—are out of luck, as both walnuts and grass are wind pollinated. But hey, if you think it works, don't let me stop you from supporting your local beekeeper.

Where I draw the line, however, is honey-infused bandages. I know honey has anti-microbial properties, but there are other critters—non-microbial ones—that like honey. They say "Don't knock it 'till you try it." Well, not me. The image of waking up to a line of ants scuttling up my leg to gnaw on a sweet-tasting bandage that is supposed to be protecting a scrape on my knee just gives me the heebie jeebies.

Allergy Season

A natural remedy for hayfever is to drink a nettle leaf and elderberry flower tea starting in early February and extending through the end of snot season, which for me is the first week of May, give or take. And I must admit, it did help. For a couple years in a row, I scooped a couple tablespoons of the

1:1 dried mixture into a large tea ball which I then dunked into a quart of freshly-boiled water. I drank a couple quarts a week. The first year I did it, I used the internet to order my ingredients in bulk. Sadly, while both nettle and elderberry can be easily found growing wild within two miles of my home, my online purchase came to me via the good folks in Hungary and Bulgaria. But I had my reasons.

I have done my fair share of "wild crafting" edible greens. It is a good idea in concept, and certainly a neat way to impress fellow hikers, kids, or a date. But for all practical purposes, there is a reason why cultivated greens are cultivated. Of the wild edibles mentioned in Wolfgang Rougle's *Sacramento Valley Feast!*, I have sampled dandelion (bitter), milk thistle (spiky), purslane (slimy), wild mustard (aphidy), chickweed (tiny), shepherd's purse (very tiny), and dock (leathery).[1] Two plants that I have gathered in large amounts are lamb's quarters, a very common weed in the spinach family, and the tangy, spade-leaved sheep sorrel. While both are nutritious and easily found and identified, a full plastic grocery bag of each always seems to cook down to less than a cup's worth of side dish. Steamed nettle leaves, while delicious (I think they taste like a delicate spinach), seem to cook down even more. And with nettle, of course, comes the obvious challenge of gathering a wild green that has a tendency to bite you before you bite it. Trying to collect and dry enough nettle to get me through the allergy season is out of the question.

As far as the elderberry flowers are concerned, the cruel joke is that cream-colored elderberry blossoms always seem to peak two weeks after my hay fever subsides, so collecting this plant requires 10 months of advanced planning. The necessity of such foresight does not play to the strength of most men in general, and me especially. But one year I endeavored to keep at least some Eastern European elderberry flowers from immigrating to Chico. I made two separate forays to collect local blossoms, filling a large kitchen-size trash bag each time. On my first attempt, there was a three-day delay between collecting the flowers and removing them from the bag. The resulting moldy plant matter might have been useful to treat some type of ailment, but it was no longer fit for hay fever tea. On my second

---
1. The one native wild green that does consistently make my happy list is miner's lettuce. When in season, it can be gathered relatively quickly and eaten raw in a salad.

try I was more diligent, and upon returning from my flower collecting adventure I quickly moved the material to a four-tray screened-in mesh drier that I hung from the clothesline. This yielded two cups of dried flowers, sprinkled with a seasoning of desiccated beetles, aphids, and other six-legged crunchies. Not the tea I was looking for.

Parting Thoughts

- Gargling warm salt water with lemon juice does wonders in relieving a sore throat.

- Wild, edible mushrooms contain lots of healthy nutrients, until your body communicates to you that a particular mushroom actually wasn't edible as you thought it was and you spend half the night puking.

- Drinking a quart of elderflower and nettle leaf tea each day made me need to pee a lot, however, its efficacy in warding off seasonal hay fever was mediocre at best.

- Love-in-a-mist seeds are NOT a cure for COVID.

- A warm mug of homemade chicken broth may or may not be the greatest medicine in the world, but it certainly tastes good.

- If your kid's feet stink, tell them to keep their shoes on in the car.

CHAPTER 7

Kettle Chips Are My Kryptonite

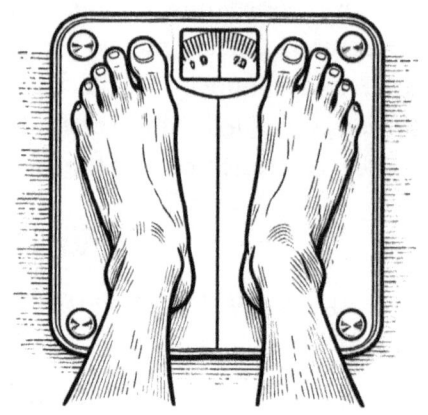

I am planning my meals for the day. It starts with six ounces of cooked oatmeal for breakfast. I will mix in a sliced banana, two ounces of nuts, a dash of salt, and a side of two large fried eggs. Lunch will be a salad that consists of greens, cut fresh veggies, and sauerkraut totaling ten ounces. I will add to this a half of an avocado (two ounces), five ounces of chopped up leftover hamburger, and a splash each of olive oil and vinegar. Lunch will conclude with four small kiwi fruit from the backyard. Dinner will be similar to lunch, but without the fruit: ten ounces of mixed, colorful vegetables (raw or cooked), five ounces of protein, and two ounces of fat—probably the other half of the avocado. My electric kitchen scale, which is sensitive down to an eighth of an ounce, has been my colleague for the past 92 days. Tomorrow, I will bid it farewell, or good riddance, depending on my mood. But this story actually begins at the other end of the gastronomical spectrum.

Picture, if you would, a donut.

Not just any donut. This is a donut drizzled with maple frosting and topped with two shimmering strips of greasy bacon. Do an internet search and you will find it. And it looks really good, even on the computer screen. For some, simply considering this image makes them salivate: sugar, fat, and salt—the holy trinity of flavor—all in one bite. We are hardwired by millennia of evolution and genetics to crave this trio because just a few thousand years ago, those humans who could access a combination of foods that were sweet, greasy, or salty had a better chance of surviving.

Of course, one does not come across a maple bacon donut every day. The same cannot be said of potato chips, which are found conveniently (and temptingly) in pretty much every checkout aisle of every supermarket, gas station, and drug store in the country. Kettle chips are my kryptonite. My primal Fred Flintstone self will always crave salted kettle-style potato chips, though the modern-day 52-year-old me realizes that my chances of enjoying a long, happy, healthy life will likely be improved if they are absent from my diet.

The Centenarian Decathlon

When considering "quality of life" over the long haul, author, podcaster, and physician Peter Attia calls upon us to consider getting our bodies in shape for the "Centenarian Decathlon." Specifically, he suggests a list of physical activities that we still might want to be able to do in our golden years and recommends that we should start "training" now, with the hope that we will extend the duration of our physical (and mental) quality of life and perhaps even have a shot of reaching the age of 100 with something left in the tank.

This is my endgame, a goal which far outpaces my desire for a daily bag of potato chips or similar snack. It is also my "now" game, for it follows that if I am currently doing what it takes to feel pretty good at 82 or even 92, then I am likely feeling *really* good at 52. In what activities might we wish to engage when we are 80 or 90 years old? Attia proposes the following Centenarian Decathlon "events," in no particular order: pick up your grandchildren (or perhaps great grandchildren); lift a carryon suitcase into an overhead airplane compartment; hike with a 20-pound backpack for an hour; get up from the floor under your own power; have sex; open a jar. To personalize this list and round it out to a neat ten, I would add: manage a #9 cast iron pan, tend a small garden, and control a medium-sized dog.

In order to achieve these goals, the usual strategies are called for: get consistent exercise and a solid night's sleep, prioritize mental and emotional health, and have mindfulness towards what foods and beverages you put into your body. I am working on the first three; however, this chapter focuses on the latter.

Where NOT to Look for a Guide to Healthy Eating

Eating is social yet personal: it can be celebratory or mundane, fast or slow, nourishing or pathological. For some it is deeply spiritual, for others it is medically restricted. For everyone it is a biological necessity. The questions are: what should we eat, when, and how much?

It is really, really, hard to find a healthy relationship with food. We are buffeted (or I should say, "buffet'd") by the food industry telling us what our eating preferences should be, and then food is designed to fit those preferences, usually with some combination of sugar (real or artificial), fat, and salt at the heart of every product. The messages about what food "should be" are as mixed as the menu of a Chinese-American restaurant at a Midwestern truck stop: food should be convenient and cheap (think McDonalds, et al.). Food is a competition (think Nathan's Hot Dog Eating contest). Food is the enemy—it makes you fat, and our society values thin, so count your calories (or scarf some Ozempic). Food should be raw. Food should be fermented. Food should be seasonal, fairly traded, high fiber, low fat, low carb, grain free, dairy free, and sugar free. There are superfoods, energy shakes, rainforest friendly foods (that froggy symbol), keto-friendly diets, and everything in between.

We are also influenced by our culture—think pasta, pupusas, curry, or kimchi—and of course by our parents, who were also guided by both culture and, if they are part of the U.S. baby-boomer generation or younger, the food industry.

Our government is not always our ally either.[1] The base of the "Food Guide Pyramid," which was promoted by the USDA from 1992-2005, depicted the ideal American diet as being supported by a variety of refined[2] foods,

---

1. It is no secret that the food industry devotes significant resources toward influencing government policies related to food and nutrition.

2. I define a refined food as any food that has been ground up or pulverized to the point where you can no longer tell what it was. While there is some grey area, like nut butter, all flours fall into this category for me.

including bread, crackers, and pasta. We were instructed to use fats and oils sparingly. The agency's current graphic, "MyPlate," doesn't even mention fats and oils, but it does highlight dairy—most commonly in the form of a beverage—as an essential part of our meal. Based on the diagram, one would assume about 15-20% of our calories (or perhaps the image refers to the weight of the food?) should come from items such as cheese, yogurt, or milk. We are told this is important to build strong bones. A catchy advertising campaign featuring a parade of smiling milk-mustachioed celebrities told my generation that milk "does a body good."

Other cultures would take exception to this. For example, dairy is not very common in Japanese cuisine—much of the population is lactose-intolerant—and yet the Japanese live longer and have lower rates of osteoporosis than in the United States. Why? Perhaps it's because they do a better job eating their green veggies. According to nutrition data from the USDA, ounce for ounce, kale, collards, spinach, and arugula all contain more calcium than milk. Broccoli, bok choy, chard, okra, and yard-long beans are not too far behind. Lamb's quarters—a common edible weed in my yard that is a distant cousin to spinach—packs nearly two and half times as much calcium as moo juice.

It can be stated that even general care medical practitioners are lacking in knowledge of how food fuels and sustains the very bodies that they are trained to heal. A survey of medical schools conducted by the Nutrition in Medicine Project at the University of North Carolina, Chapel Hill, found that as of 2004, only 40 of 104 institutions (38%) met the minimum 25 required hours of nutrition education set by the National Academy of Sciences.

Fifteen years later this reality did not appear to have changed much. As pointed out by *Time* magazine, a 2021 survey of medical schools in the U.S. and U.K., published in the *Journal of Human Nutrition and Dietetics*, found that most students receive an average of 11 hours of nutrition training throughout an entire medical program. Part of this training is typically student-run. John Robbins, author of *Diet for a New America* and *The Food Revolution* accurately summarizes the gravity of this concern when he quips: "A doctor who doesn't know about food is like a firefighter who doesn't know about water."

Despite All of This, We All Need to Eat

My own food journey actually got off to a pretty good start. My dad maintained a robust veggie garden, so as a young kid growing up in the 1970s foods such as chard, zucchini, cherry tomatoes, and green beans all made frequent appearances at the dinner table. My mother made sure that a green vegetable was always present (even if my brother and I didn't always eat it). My family also enjoyed an abundance of seasonal fruit from the trees in our yard, including peaches, plums, and apricots. Generally speaking, Safeway supplied the rest of our food, and my mom came home with paper grocery bags containing items such as Fleischman's margarine, canned creamed corn, Campbell's Chunky Soup, Lender's Bagels, Honey Nut Cheerios, cardboard canisters of frozen orange juice, boxes of Kraft Mac & Cheese, fish sticks, tater tots, ground beef, iceberg lettuce, tin roof sundae ice cream, frozen lima beans, and plenty of milk.

This typical 1980s diet gave me plenty of energy to grow big and strong, giving me the endurance to watch endless hours of television, and at the same time bike up to two miles to school each day and participate in ten-mile hikes and 50-mile backpacking trips with my Boy Scout troop. The problem was, I was also short, barely reaching five feet at the conclusion of middle school. By the time I became a peach-fuzz lipped, acne-faced high school sophomore, I had the build of a diminutive offensive lineman—the guys that look like they could be sumo wrestler crossovers. A year into college, after having indulged in more than my fair share of lasagna and chicken strips from the food service buffet troughs, I was, well, a pretty wide boy. This despite being an avid participant in intramural sports and spending a few hours a week in the gym.

David Asprey, author of the book *Game Changers*, found himself in a similar situation, and recognized that exercise alone can take you so far:

> In my experience, when people focus too much on the idea of exercise, they often waste a lot of time and effort. When I weighed 300 pounds, I resolved to exercise my way out of it. I worked out for ninety minutes a day six days a week for eighteen months. No matter how much it hurt or how tired I was, every day I did forty-five minutes of cardio and forty-five minutes of weight training. The

demotivating (and demoralizing) result was that I ended up being a very strong obese person.

I also considered myself pretty strong. Tired of being called chubby, in my late teens I responded by practicing what I called "inverted pushups," where I did a handstand against the wall and proceeded to raise and lower my body using my arms. At one point I could do twenty. But I was still overweight. And I was still called chubby.

Until this time, my relationship with food had been a combination of functional and impulsive. Influenced by the fast pace of college, food was something to be shoveled into one's mouth and perhaps be enjoyed in the process, but my connection with it didn't go much further. And it showed, most notably on the scale, and also in the mirror. I did not like what I saw. So midway through my second year of college, I made a conscious decision to change my relationship with food. I decided that food was now the enemy, something to be kept at arm's length. For the next six months I stopped eating dairy, sweets, and seconds. I cut out red meat to follow the eco-recommendation of eating lower on the food chain, and because I thought it was better for the planet (which it likely is) and better for my health (which it likely wasn't). I kept myself distracted with sports and classes. I nearly passed out (twice) and was borderline anorexic.

I lost over 30 pounds that spring and began a weight gain-weight loss yo-yo that would continue for the next twenty years. I held active jobs in my twenties and early thirties that helped me successfully process much of the "crap food" that I put into my body, including such delicacies as French fries or corn nuts, washed down with a Snapple pink lemonade. Then came more sedentary employment as a classroom teacher, followed by parenthood and the sense of obligation that I needed to finish any of the food left on my young daughter's plate. The bathroom mirror revealed a slow transformation to the iconic dad-bod. Increasing stiffness in my lower back followed.

Goodbye Dairy. Farewell Gluten.

Things started to change in the winter of 2011, when my family's evening routine began to include the following words from our toddler: "Mommy,

Daddy—My tummy hurts." This was often accompanied by an after-hours bout of mucus-dominated pukage. We determined that our daughter was frequently congested in the evening, and soon after going to bed this excess of phlegm would work its way into her stomach, causing nausea. A naturopath inquired as to how much dairy we ate. At the time, dairy was indeed a substantial part of our family's diet. I recall whole milk mozzarella cheese as being a main staple. It was suggested that we try eliminating milk products for a few weeks to see what happens. Well, problem solved.

A couple years later, our intake of gluten-containing products met with a similar fate. My wife had struck up a conversation with the preschool teacher about healthy eating and her personal challenges with digestion, which led to a suggestion that she take a break from gluten, an experiment that was adopted by the whole family. The effect was more than notable. Not only did my wife start feeling better, but daughter's eczema slowly began to clear, and my chronic back pain began to ease.

Many doctors would not be surprised that eliminating gluten could be linked to such a range of healing. A growing body of research is demonstrating that, for many, gluten triggers inflammation ranging from skin maladies (such as eczema), to irritable bowel, to aching joints (such as backs).

I also got sick less—a lot less. And when I did get sick, I found that I recovered faster—colds, sniffles, sore throats, you name it—even as I spent extended time in classrooms with first-year college students (not the healthiest group when a virus is going through the dorms), not to mention the germs that my kids brought home from preschool and kindergarten.

An additional effect of eliminating gluten was that we also removed from our family's diet a huge source of carbohydrates, specifically those coming from refined wheat flour. Finely ground foods, be it a grain or a nut, are digested more quickly—some experts say too quickly—than "whole" nuts or grains, such as rice. Resulting spikes in glucose levels provide an energy burst followed by the post-lunch burrito coma (or pasta coma, or burger and fries coma). Generally speaking, excess carbohydrates that are not used by the body end up being stored as fat.

A Mountain of Vegetables

Inspired by a desire for our family to continue to broaden our healthy eating habits, we read. The body of literature making recommendations about the "ideal diet" is robust and seems to have exploded over the last 15 years, and my wife and I indulged. (Full disclosure: My wife listened to many of the books first on Audible, and then I read them as per her suggestions.) The reading list included works by Barbra Kingsolver (eat local), Michael Pollan (if your grandmother wouldn't recognize it, don't eat it), Robb Wolf (that Paleo guy), Dr. David Perlmutter (the "carbs are bad" guy), Dr. Terry Wahls (autoimmune conditions), Susan Pierce Thompson (sugar and flour are addictive), Weston A. Price (eat sauerkraut, liver, and nuts), and more.

Add to this the fact that my professional career as an environmental educator already had (and still has) me thinking and learning about the importance of humanity's connection—or disconnection—with its food. I frequently quip that my weekly, and sometimes biweekly, bike trips to the local farmers' markets are my version of going to church, except I come away with much more than a wafer. It is my connection not only to my food and the people who grew it, but also to my community.

As I have alluded to, I most certainly did not embark on such a food journey on my own. Credit (a LOT of credit) must be given to my wife, whose voracious appetite for information and self-betterment has paved the way for me and the rest of our family to find foods that best meet our needs. She also has an appetite for vegetables, and she leads by example. Our daughters began to refer to her dinner plate as "Mount Mommy." Her platter of chopped green veggies along with a rainbow of other plant parts regularly reaches an elevation of—no joke—over six inches above her plate. Despite her petite frame, she eats like Rabbitzilla, devouring mixed salad greens, cooked kale, bok choy, zucchini, sauerkraut, tomatoes, beets, sweet potato, bell pepper, broccoli, and yes, carrots. While my wife is not a vegetarian (though she was for 26 years), the final topper of five ounces of chopped chicken she adds often seems more like a garnish than a focal point of the meal. But hey, it works for her, and has served as a role model for the rest of us, helping us to recognize that the definition of a tasty, filling meal need not be limited to traditional American standby of beef, potatoes, and an afterthought iceberg lettuce side salad. To be blunt, my wife is a food mindfulness superhero.

So Long, Dad-Bod

At some point, I was introduced to the "Whole30" diet. To be quite honest, I didn't read much into the nuts and bolts (though I knew that nuts would be on the menu), but I felt I had a pretty good grasp of the basics: by this time, I was already minimizing my intake of dairy, refined sugars, processed foods, and gluten (my only wheat flour was from the occasional farmers' market burrito). What if I went cold turkey—100% elimination—of these foods for 30 days? How would I feel? This would be a "reset diet," a way to start with a clean slate (or perhaps a clean plate?). For me, the biggest appeal of the Whole30 diet was the time duration. I could tell myself that this was not a forever decision, but it would be a challenge, a personal "I triple-dog-dare you" for lack of better terminology. And it would also be a good science experiment, as thirty days allows enough time to actually see if a change in diet has made a difference. So, for one month (not December, thank god) I followed the plan: no grains, no sweetener of any sort, no refined foods, no legumes other than green beans and snap peas (I can't remember why), and no dairy. I paid attention to my body, taking care to separate the feelings of hunger from the more primal desire to have a flavor in my mouth (even when I wasn't hungry). As such, I snacked less. Similarly, I focused on noting the moment I found myself sated by a meal, and then I stopped eating, even if there was still food left on my plate. I reminded myself that I could always save leftovers for later. I held back from eating the kids' leftovers too, either putting them in a container into the fridge or declaring them to be treats for our chickens to be eventually transformed into fresh eggs.

At the end of the 30 days, I took stock of what changes I was ready to adopt as a permanent part of my diet. I found I had incorporated a LOT more veggies into my meals, especially greens, while at the same time I had reduced my portions of meat, and I was happy continuing to do so (good for the planet as well as my body). I also noticed I found myself less dependent on foods such as rice or oats. I was able to gauge how much food was "right" for each meal such that I got up from the dining table feeling satisfied without feeling stuffed. And while I relaxed the restrictions on many of the food limitations of the Whole30 diet, I did choose to ditch gluten entirely.

So adding it all up: less carbs from grains, zero gluten, minimal dairy, fewer refined foods, less sugar, lots of locally-grown plants, and more awareness equaled—over a ten year period—increased overall stamina, fewer creaking joints (knee, back), reduced illness, and yes, less Dad-Bod.

But . . . there were still the kettle chips, which made my way into the grocery cart on most visits. And there was also the between-meal nut and raisin grab. And the post-dinner piece of chocolate (or two) to get me through washing dishes (dark chocolate contains essential antioxidants, so I've been told, and choose to believe). And the mid-morning gluten-free muffin. And the mid-afternoon rice cake (I liked the satisfying crunch). And the occasional spoonful of peanut butter sprinkled with salt.

The Last 10 Pounds

This brings me to when I began to weigh my food.

There are a number of "diet plans" out there along with scientific studies stating that most of them really don't work. Often, the most restrictive diets tend to be the least effective, because as we know, greasy, salty, and sweet taste damn good. Author Pilar Gerasimo, in her book *The Healthy Deviant*, cites UCLA research that "suggests that all restrictive diets eventually fail and/or backfire, often leading subjects to gain back the weight they have lost, and then some." Gerasimo goes on to point out that contemporary dietary research supports the idea that the quality of one's food, rather than quantity, is what leads to the healthiest outcomes. In other words, don't count calories, but read the ingredients. She suggests "eating mostly real, whole, nutrient-dense foods and avoiding crappy, processed, addictive, inflammatory food-like products high in flours, sugars, oils, salts, and toxic additives." This was all fine and good, but my family had already done a fairly decent job checking these boxes.

With all due respect to Gerasimo, I realized that my personal biggest challenge was breaking myself of the habit of unnecessary snacking (aka eating when I wasn't hungry), which was essentially adding up to a fourth meal every day. For this I needed a plan that was up to the task, one that would make my food choices black and white, yes and no, with no b.s. Fortunately, such a diet plan exists. I will call it the "No B.S. Plan," or NBS for short. And yes, this is a real diet plan, but the acronym has been changed to protect the innocent.

What initially attracted me to NBS—besides the strong endorsement by my wife—was its no-nonsense approach to eating. That said, I feel the overall philosophy of the program does a fine job incorporating contemporary thoughts on what constitutes a healthy diet. In summary:

- It accepts the fact that carbohydrates, fats, and protein are all necessary.
- Humans were designed to eat whole, unprocessed foods without added sugars.
- Generally speaking, Americans eat more food than they need to.
- For most people, eating just three times a day is sufficient.

With all of this in mind, NBS clearly outlines what you can't have, what you can have, and how much.

So for four months, I strove to eliminate the following foods from my diet: all flour (including gluten-free flours, nut flours, and cornmeal), fruit juice, all natural and artificial sweeteners (including honey and maple syrup), rice or potatoes with any meal besides breakfast, fruit for dinner, dried fruit (source of concentrated sugar), all in-between meal snacks, and yes, even my beloved kettle chips. I weighed my food, following the program's recommendations about how many ounces of proteins, fats, grains, vegetables, and fruits I should eat at each meal. And I was hungry—not starving, but definitely hungry (and sometimes hangry)—pretty much every day.

So how does the NBS program avoid the poor track record of other highly restrictive diets? The answer: by providing participants with a TON of resources, including numerous web-based videos and documents, frequent online coaching opportunities, and actively facilitating and supporting participation in a robust online community. I was impressed. If your culture informs how you eat, then having a diet program that provides a supportive community of like-minded individuals makes a lot of sense. And so once again, I hit the reset button and made a pact with myself to stick to the plan, taking stock at the end of every month to see where I was at, and if I wanted to continue. This time, however, I started on November 5, and punched the diet train through the culinary minefield of an East Coast wedding, Thanksgiving, my birthday, my two daughters' birthdays, and the December holidays.

It was brutal.

"Everything in Moderation. Including Moderation" ~ Oscar Wilde

I think the most difficult moment was the ice cream. My younger daughter's "double scoop" from the downtown ice cream shop was actually a quadruple-scoop bounty, far more than she could eat. Coconut ice cream over a mango sorbet. I was a cool month and half into my "eating plan," having limited my sweet treat indulgences during this time to a single polite sliver of my mom's pumpkin chiffon pie at Thanksgiving and a bourbon barrel-aged stout on my birthday. I stared and stared at my daughter's half-eaten dessert. I could have saved the excess ice cream from the trash bin, but I was "good." And it was *damn* tough.

My two goals had been to drop ten pounds and to change my eating habits such that I could keep it off as part of my "training regimen" for the Centenarian Decathlon. (Or, if I did end up gaining weight, I wanted it to be gained from muscle mass.) That said, I had no desire to add misery to my life by abstaining from delicious food for the rest of my years. Would eating ice cream every now and again truly impact my ability to free-weight future grandchildren? Didn't I read that longevity is also correlated with happiness? What's the point of hefting Junior if you aren't able to smile in the process? The question is, if finishing off my daughter's ice cream once a month makes me happier, will I live longer?

According to one oft-cited study published in the *British Medical Journal*, the answer is "Yes." The researchers surveyed a cohort of Harvard alumni and found that those who ate candy one to three times a month were likely to add as much as a year to their life as compared to non-candy consumers.

While the study did not describe what types of candy the participants were eating, one speculates that if you are limiting your indulgences to just once every week or two, then those moments are really enjoyed. My takeaway: while eating five pieces of Halloween candy a day for all of November and December is not advised, if the occasional scoop of gelato makes you happy, then go for it because happier people live longer.

The Last 3 Pounds

It just ain't going to happen. I dropped six pounds in the first month. The seventh pound took another month. And now? Seventy days into my kettle chip moratorium I believe it is an appropriate time for excuses and reflection ("rexcuses?" "excution?"). Perhaps my body is now the weight it is "meant to be." Perhaps I have been exercising more that I had thought, and denser muscle is replacing more buoyant fat (come to think of it, I am finding myself getting cold more easily). Perhaps my bathroom scale is jammed.

It is also possible that I have reached a new "set point weight" by practicing *"hara hachi bun me,"* a Confucian teaching that instructs people to eat until they are 80 percent full. A related Japanese proverb acknowledges the value of avoiding overeating: "Eight parts of a full stomach sustain the man; the other two sustain the doctor." Nevertheless, up to three times a day my inner caveman keeps telling me that I am 20% short of feeling truly sated, and he is not happy about it.

I have drunk many cups of creatively-flavored herbal teas over the past few months, trying to trick my body into thinking it was a snack. My stomach is not so easily fooled.

The Last Pound, aka "Good Enough"

Ninety days of NBS, nine pounds lost. I am calling it good enough and declaring that I am done. Not because I think NBS is wrong or that it doesn't work, but because I don't think I need it anymore—I have succeeded in my primary goal, which is kicking my in-between meal and late-night snacking habits. My mantras: hunger is not an emergency, and there is always another meal just a few hours (or a night's sleep) away. I am also pleased with much of the gastronomic re-awakening I have been able to experience. For example, the sweetness of in-season, locally-grown fresh fruit never tasted so good, and I have a new favorite breakfast, a true "break the fast" after going up to 15 hours without eating: Farmers' Market sweet potato with black beans, topped with two fried eggs, a healthy dollop of salsa, a handful of raw pumpkin seeds, a couple shakes of salt and a piece of seasonal fruit on the side.

That said, I am ready to allow myself the occasional treat, such as finishing my daughter's ice cream or enjoying some corn chips and guacamole at a Mexican restaurant while dining with friends—you know, the things that make me happy. As far as snacking, I will not deny the logic of grabbing a handful of trail mix while on a hike. I will check in with myself every six months or so to see how I am doing. I proved to myself that I can do the NBS diet once; if I deem it necessary, I can simply choose to do it again.

I consider myself fortunate in this regard. Through reading the NBS articles, listening to the vlogs and, most directly, while participating in the online NBS community by way of both text threads and Zoom meet-ups, I recognized that, for many people, NBS is both a necessary and welcomed regimen. It is well-documented that the Standard American Diet (what many dieticians refer to as the "SAD" diet) adversely affects our physical and mental health. Our country has one of the highest rates of heart disease and stroke in the world, and our collective eating habits have been singled out as the biggest culprit. Globally, a 2019 *Lancet* study affirmed that poor diet is responsible for more deaths than any other risk factor. Certainly, this is something to be aware of when you are in training to live into your 90s and beyond. Many NBS participants I spoke to told stories of friends and relatives dying young, and of doctors that pointed out that unless they made some changes in their lifestyle—especially their diet—they were on a similar path to a shortened lifespan. It doesn't help that the SAD diet is highly addictive. You know what I am talking about: salt, sugar, fat, and the ingrained survival instincts of our inner caveperson. Pavlov reigns supreme—my mouth still waters at the thought of kettle chips, my brain craves the chemical reward that comes from eating that first crunchy, salty, greasy bite, and the second, the third . . . half the bag . . .

I am lucky. I can tell myself that chips, ice cream, pasta, cookies, or candied nuts (yes, I am talking about the ones from Trader Joe's) aren't necessary, and I am surrounded by a culture and family that supports me when I choose to not eat them. For many people this is not the case. The coffee break room, the workplace holiday party, and celebratory family gatherings all include foods—and expectations to indulge—that are difficult, if not near impossible, to resist. This does not even touch on the temptations we see every day in the supermarket check-out aisle or gas station convenience store. Even the "natural foods store" is a force to be reckoned with: added sugar is added sugar, even if it comes as in the form of organic honey or maple syrup used as sweetener in a bulk purchase of locally-crafted granola. For many, "It tastes so good" all too quickly crosses the line to addiction. To counter these realities, NBS participants have embraced the rigid rules of the NBS "maintenance diet" every day with zeal, and they lean on coaches and other participants for support as needed.

We Are What We Eat

I took a road trip with a friend a few years ago, and the question arose of where to stop for lunch. We were on the interstate; the options were plentiful. I suggested we pick up Subway sandwiches. The response from my comrade was quick and emphatic: "No, not Subway."

Huh? In my mind this was a perfectly reasonable option—Subway was inexpensive, highly accessible, and an improvement (so I thought at the time) over the traditional fast-food establishments advertised by red, orange, or yellow signage (hard-earned scientific research has determined that the colors red, orange, and yellow make us hungry). My friend continued: "Have you ever noticed what it smells like in a Subway Sandwich shop?"

"Sure, it smells like a Subway Sandwich Shop"

"That's my point. They serve sandwiches. It should smell like a *delicatessen*."

This gave me pause. He was quite right. A delicatessen smells like sourdough or pumpernickel rye bread made with six ingredients or less. It smells like large hunks of smoked turkey and roast beef and pastrami and provolone cheese ready to be cut to order. It smells like soup of the day, spicy mustard, and half-sour pickles. It smells like lunch.

Subway smells like a voluminous tub of mayonnaise, school-lunch potato chip bags, and clonal rows of chemically perfected 17-ingredient "Artisan Italian (white) Bread."

Whether by intention or ignorance, all too often we either do not know, or we do not care to know, what we are putting into our bodies. While we are aware, at some level, that packaged junk food contains dozens of ingredients that are not easily identifiable as "food," we eat it anyway. Author Michael Pollan recommends that we abstain from ingesting that which we cannot pronounce. Perhaps the greater challenge is when wholesome-looking food turns out not to be wholesome. We may overindulge too frequently, or we don't recognize when a product contains excess sugar, or we aren't fully cognizant of our own body's response—both in the short term and the long term—to eating processed foods. Similarly, we are oblivious of the journey that food takes to get to our plates: the quality of the soil in the corn field, the working conditionings of the farmer or factory worker, the energy or water footprint of our meal, or the other numerous resources that it takes to grow, package, and distribute our lunch, not to mention the systems in place to facilitate the disposal of any packaging or food waste.

How can we have a relationship with our food if we don't even know what our food is? So here is my final nugget of dietary advice. Clearly identify what foods you are placing into your body, and then go out and find the relationship with those foods that works for you. They say that we are what we eat. If this is true, then perhaps it can be argued that our society has an identity crisis.

How can we know who we are, if we don't even know what we are eating?

CHAPTER 8

Feed Your Soul

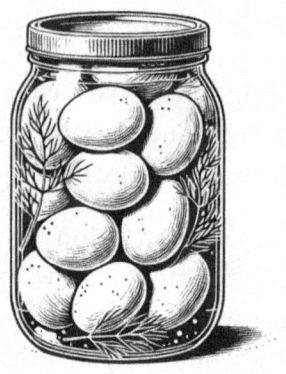

Someday I may write a full-fledged recipe book with my family's favorite dishes. But for now, the sampling that appears on the following pages will have to suffice. In our home, we try to emphasize colorful seasonal and local fruits and vegetables, whole grains and amazing flavors while downplaying dairy and refined sugar. Our recipes tend to be simple and nourishing. *Bon appetit!*

Almond Milk

I used to purchase this from the Farmers' Market until I learned how easy it is to make. Use as you would regular milk—in coffee, breakfast cereal, or baking. Yields just over a quart.

Ingredients:

    1 cup raw almonds

    4 cups water

Directions:

1. Soak almonds in water overnight in the refrigerator.
2. Drain water and rinse almonds.
3. Add four cups of fresh water to a blender.
4. Add almonds to the blender.
5. Blend on high for 2 minutes.
6. Strain milk through a fine strainer and capture in a large bowl (I use an organic cotton bag made by EcoPeaceful (www.ecopeaceful.com). Squeeze or press the almond meal to get as much milk as you can.
7. Store milk in a 1-quart jar in the fridge, use within four days.
8. Freeze almond meal for later use in baking recipes.

Carrot Cake Muffins

Gluten free, dairy free, and freezable—this treat checks off a lot of boxes. Use less honey if your carrots are really sweet or you are using dried cranberries (which usually have added sugar). Makes ~16 muffins, which can be served with breakfast or as a dessert.

Ingredients:

- 3 large eggs
- ¼ cup coconut oil
- 1 cup almond flour or almond meal (I use the leftover meal from making almond milk)
- 1 cup oat flour (I make my own as needed by grinding dry rolled oats in a small electric coffee grinder)
- 1/3 to ½ cup of honey, depending on sweetness preference
- 1 cup shredded carrots
- ½ cup chopped walnuts or pecans
- ½ cup raisins or dried cranberries
- 1 tsp cinnamon
- ½ tsp nutmeg
- ½ tsp ginger powder
- ¼ tsp salt
- ½ tsp baking soda
- ½ tsp baking powder
- 1 tsp vanilla extract
- 4 oz (~ ½ cup) apple sauce
- 2 tbsp water

Directions:

1. Preheat oven to 350F degrees.
2. Mix all dry ingredients in a large bowl: Almond meal, nuts, raisins or cranberries, spices, baking soda, baking powder, salt.
3. Use a fork to whip three eggs until uniform color.

4. Melt coconut oil (if solid), mix with honey, water, applesauce, vanilla and eggs.
5. Combine all ingredients into the large bowl, add carrots and mix.
6. Place into muffin cups in a muffin tin.
7. Bake for ~30 minutes.
8. Let cool. Eat some fresh, share or freeze the rest. Goes especially well with cream cheese or butter.

Gado Gado

This dish is essentially steamed seasonal vegetables over rice served with a Southeast Asian style sauce. Its simplicity, combined with the sheer diversity of vegetable options makes it a winner for my family. Tofu or hard-boiled eggs are included for additional protein. The sauce recipe includes 3 tablespoons of brown sugar, but you can choose to reduce the sugar or omit it entirely.

Sauce:

    1 cup peanut of almond butter
    1 tbsp grated ginger
    1 tbsp coarsely chopped garlic
    3 tbsp brown sugar
    1½ cups hot water
    4 tbsp apple cider vinegar
    2 tbsp soy sauce
    1 tsp salt
    Crushed red pepper to taste

Blend all ingredients until sauce is uniform in texture and color. Serve as a dressing warm or cold. Leftovers can be stored in the refrigerator.

Rice:

    2 cups short-grained white rice
    3 ¼ cups water
    ½ tsp turmeric powder

1. Combine all ingredients in a pot, bring the pot to a boil.
2. Simmer with the lid on until all water is absorbed.

Vegetables/Toppings:

Any of the following can be steamed; choose among them based on personal preference and seasonality. I usually cook 6 to 8 different items, filling the steamer. Eggs are hard boiled separately. A diversity of colors is recommended. Slicing directions are suggestions only. Leftovers can be stored in the refrigerator.

- Zucchini, sliced into ½ inch thick rounds or 3" long spears
- Yellow summer squash sliced into ½ inch rounds or 3" long spears
- Red onion, sliced into 8 wedges
- Green onion, 4" lengths
- Potato, ½ inch slices
- Daikon radish, ½ inch thick rounds or 3-inch-long spears
- Broccoli florets
- Cauliflower florets
- Red cabbage wedges
- Red radishes, halved
- Snow peas
- Green beans (or purple or yellow)
- Carrot, sliced at a 45-degree angle into ½ inch thick ellipses
- Celery, sliced at a 45-degree angle in ¾ inch thick chunks
- Bell pepper, any color, seeded and sliced into 6 to 8 pieces
- Beet, sliced into wedges
- Firm tofu, 1" cubes
- Hard boiled eggs, peeled

Present steamed veggies, tofu and eggs on a large tray, platter, or lasagna dish. Serve plates or bowls of rice and allow each guest to use tongs to select toppings as desired. Sauce is added last. Can also be served with soy sauce.

Brown Rice Salad

This recipe comes from Glenn County organic rice farmer Greg Massa, with a few minor tweaks. It is a great potluck dish. You can try substituting cilantro for the parsley, or adding in some fresh chopped mint leaves.

Ingredients:

    2 cups short-grain brown rice, uncooked
    1 cup raisins or pomegranate seeds
    Zest of 1 orange
    3 tbsp olive oil
    1 bunch parsley, chopped
    ¾ cup pecans
    Juice of 1 orange
    Salt and pepper to taste
    Optional: crumbled feta or goat cheese
    Optional: grated carrot, enough to add color

Directions:

1. Cook rice as per instructions, allow to cool completely.
2. Combine all ingredients, refrigerate for at least one hour prior to serving.

Ratatouille

This is an excellent way to use a lot of fresh summer veggies in a single, one pot dish. Can be served over rice, polenta, or pasta, or on its own as a chunky stew. Vary the amounts of each ingredient with joyful fearlessness based on preference and availability. Leftovers are awesome, the flavor gets stronger after a couple days in the fridge. I usually double the recipe, and triple the amount of summer squash.

Ingredients:

    3 tbsp olive oil
    4 medium garlic cloves, finely chopped
    2 cups chopped onion
    1 bay leaf
    1 medium Italian eggplant, cut into 1" cubes
    1½ tsp salt
    1½ tsp dried basil or 3 tbsp fresh, chopped
    1 tsp dried oregano or 1 tbsp fresh, chopped
    ½ tsp rosemary
    ½ tsp dried thyme or ½ tbsp fresh
    1 medium zucchini or other summer squash, cubed
    2 medium bell peppers, coarsely chopped
    14.5 oz canned tomatoes, or 4 medium fresh, cut into large chunks
    Optional: 1 cup chopped Greek olives
    Optional: 1-2 lbs of sweet or spicy Italian sausage, cut into chunks

Directions:

1. In a large pot or saucepan, sauté garlic and onion in olive oil for five minutes.
2. Add eggplant, salt, and herbs. Cook on medium heat for 15-20 minutes or until eggplant is soft.
3. Add remaining ingredients. Simmer on low heat until all vegetables are tender.
4. Serve hot over rice, pasta, or polenta, or serve on its own as a hot or cold stew.

Gazpacho

Originating from Spain and Portugal, I consider gazpacho to be a cousin to ratatouille in that it is very flavorful and takes advantage of a lot of fresh summer vegetables, especially cucumbers and tomatoes. It is extremely easy to prepare, and can be served as a cold soup or used liberally as a salsa. Some gazpacho recipes incorporate bread crusts, but we prefer ours without. Feel free to vary the amounts of veggies as you see fit. I usually include the basil leaves, forgo the tomato juice, and double the recipe.

Ingredients:

- 1 large green cucumber or 3 yellow "lemon" cucumbers
- 4 medium size juicy tomatoes
- 2 red bell peppers, seeded
- 1 red onion
- 3 garlic cloves
- ¼ cup white wine vinegar
- ¼ cup olive oil
- ½ tbsp salt
- 1 tsp black pepper
- Cayenne powder to taste
- Optional: Handful of fresh basil leaves
- Optional: Add tomato juice to make more juicy (though using fresh tomatoes is usually sufficient)

Directions:

1. Coarsely chop all vegetables.
2. Mix all ingredients in a large bowl.
3. Blend in batches to desired consistency, using a blender or food processor.
4. Serve cold.

Sauerkraut

We use sauerkraut liberally as a dinner condiment, with its salty tangy flavor adding character to meat and rice. Feel free to experiment, but toss out any batches that develop a pink color or smells like anything other than cabbage, sauerkraut, or other strong-scented inclusions (such as garlic).

Beginners should avoid using red or purple vegetables such as beets, red cabbage or purple carrots, as these will stain your batch making it harder to detect contamination.

This recipe makes 3 quarts of sauerkraut, which can be stored in the fridge for four to six months. If you wish, you can reduce the total amount of vegetables, but I recommend that the cabbage remain at least 75% of the total weight, and keep the salt to vegetable ratio the same (1 tbsp salt for 2 lbs vegetables). There are lots of ways to set up your sauerkraut ferment, this is just the one that I have found works best for me.

Ingredients:

- 4.5 lbs green cabbage, chopped or shredded
- 1.5 lbs of other vegetables, good options include carrot spears, daikon radish spears, small cauliflower florets, and garlic cloves (I do not recommend exceeding 15 large cloves)
- 3 tbsp non-iodized salt

Directions:

1. Combine your vegetables in a large bowl.
2. Mix in the salt.
3. Cover the bowl with a large towel (as you would cover bread dough that is left to rise) and let sit at room temperature for 45 – 60 minutes.
4. Place the entire contents of the bowl into a clean 1-gallon glass jar (or similar). Stuff in vegetables using clean fists, packing it as tight as possible. Be sure to include any liquid at the bottom of the bowl. Wide-mouth quart jars can also be used, 6 pounds of vegetables will require four jars, with the material divided evenly

between them. There should be at least two inches of space left in the top of the jar(s).

5. Fill a 1-gallon Ziplock bag about 1/3 with water and then seal the bag, taking care to remove as much air as possible. (Use quart-size bags if using quart jars). Place the bag in the jar on top of the cabbage, such that the shape of the bag fills the remaining space in the top of the jar. Try to massage the bag such that there are minimal pockets of air between the bag and the cabbage (a little air is OK). You can carefully add or remove water from the Ziplock as needed, resealing it when you are done.

6. Put the entire jar in a large bowl or round platter with a side, such as a circular cake pan. This is to contain any liquid that spills out from the top of the jar during the period of fermentation (similar to a tray beneath a flower pot for capturing excess water). This liquid will likely get moldy, but that's okay, it will eventually be discarded.

7. Place the tray and the jar in an out-of-the way location where it can remain at room temperature.

8. After 14–21 days (longer will yield a more tangy flavor), gently bring the sauerkraut jar to the sink. You can take the jar out of the tray at this time and pour any excess liquid from the tray down the drain.

9. Carefully remove the bag and wipe the rim of the jar of any cabbage pieces that might have been exposed to the air. The contents should smell like sauerkraut, and be free of any pink coloring.

10. Using tongs and a canning funnel, fill three clean wide-mouth quart jars with the sauerkraut, evening dividing any liquid. Add a lid to each jar and store in the refrigerator for four to six months.

Pickled Eggs

My older daughter insisted this recipe be included. It is a simplified version of directions I received from Samantha Zangrilli of Turkey Tail Farm. After two weeks, the eggs achieve a consistency of slightly tangy cheese, and can be enjoyed as a high-protein snack or as a salad topper. Leftover brine makes a fine dressing when paired with olive or avocado oil.

Ingredients:

- 11 hard-boiled eggs, peeled
- ¾ cups cider vinegar
- ¾ cups water
- ½ tbsp salt
- 6 large garlic cloves, crushed
- 1/3 cup packed fresh dill or basil, coarsely chopped (or 1 rounded tablespoon of dried dill or basil)
- 1-quart wide-mouth jar, with a lid

Directions:

1. Gently place the eggs into the jar, leaving room for all the eggs to be fully immersed in liquid (depending on the size of your eggs, it is possible that only nine or ten will fit).
2. In a small pot, combine the water, vinegar, salt, garlic, and basil and bring to a boil. Stir until all the salt is dissolved.
3. Allow the liquid to cool for a minute.
4. Pour the liquid into the jar, making sure all the herbs have been included. Fill until the eggs are covered, and then discard any extra liquid that doesn't fit.
5. Cover the jar with a lid, and allow to cool before placing into the refrigerator.
6. Allow eggs to cure for at least two weeks. Keep refrigerated. Consume within three months.

Moroccan-Style Spice Mix

I multiply the amounts listed by a factor of 8 to make roughly 2 cups of spice mix, which is stored in a jar in the cupboard. We use it liberally as a flavoring for lamb, chicken, and salmon.

1 teaspoon each of:

- Ginger powder
- Cumin powder
- Turmeric powder
- Paprika powder
- Garlic powder
- Red pepper flakes

½ tsp each of:

- Cinnamon powder
- Coriander powder
- Nutmeg powder
- Clove powder
- Finely ground black pepper

1½ tsp salt

Latke Waffles

A family take on a Jewish holiday favorite; they can be enjoyed throughout the year for any meal. Latkes are traditionally a potato pancake fried in olive oil, but we switched to the waffle iron because it is less messy and looks cool. This version is gluten free. Optional add-ins are included, feel free to be creative. Makes about sixteen 4 x 4-inch waffles. Note: Do NOT use a Belgium-style waffle iron, the pits are too deep.

Ingredients:

- 2.5 lbs potatoes, grated (if using brown-skinned Russets I recommend peeling them)
- 1 small white or yellow onion, diced
- 2 large eggs
- 1.5 tsp salt
- ¼ cup potato starch or potato flour
- Olive oil spray
- Optional vegetables to consider adding (replaces up to one potato): diced greens, such as kale, chard, spinach, or parsley; grated cauliflower, broccoli stem, or kohlrabi; grated winter squash; diced zucchini or bell peppers
- Optional spices to consider (fresh or dried): garlic, paprika, black pepper, chili powder, basil, thyme, oregano

Directions:

1. Grate the potatoes. Squeeze the liquid into a separate bowl and set aside, place the grated potato into a large mixing bowl.
2. Dice the onion. Add onions, eggs, salt, and potato starch to the bowl.
3. By now there should be additional potato starch that has settled to the bottom of the bowl of liquid you set aside. Drain off the liquid and add the potato starch to the bowl.
4. Mix all ingredients thoroughly.
5. Allow waffle iron to heat up. Spray the bottom griddle with olive oil, and add a small dollop (about ½ cup) of batter to each

section. Spray the top of each dollop with a short spritz of olive oil, close the waffle iron, and use an oven mitt to gently press the iron down.

6. Cooking time is 5 to 10 minutes, depending on the temperature of your waffle maker. Traditionally served with sour cream and applesauce.